NURSING ASSISTANT
REVIEW
FOR COMPETENCY EVALUATION

Second Edition

Sheila A. Sorrentino, RN, PhD

CherylAnn S. Owoc, RN, BSN, MEd

with 12 illustrations

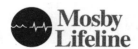

Mosby
Lifeline

St. Louis Baltimore Boston Carlsbad Chicago Naples New York Philadelphia Portland
London Madrid Mexico City Singapore Sydney Tokyo Toronto Wiesbaden

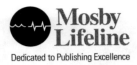

Mosby Lifeline
Dedicated to Publishing Excellence

A Times Mirror Company

Vice President and Publisher: David Dusthimer
Managing Editor: Doris E. Smith
Assistant Editor: Elaine M. Wilburt
Project Manager: Chris Baumle
Production Editor: David Orzechowski
Book Design: Nancy McDonald

Printed in the United States of America
Composition by Monotype Composition Company, Inc.
Printing/binding by Plus Communications

Mosby–Year Book, Inc.
11830 Westline Industrial Drive
St. Louis, Missouri 63146

ISBN 0-8151-8625-8
96 97 98 99 00/ 9 8 7 6 5 4 3 2 1

NURSING ASSISTANT
REVIEW
FOR COMPETENCY EVALUATION

This book is dedicated to the certified nursing assistants. Each day you enhance the quality of your residents' lives through your professionalism, respect for residents' rights, and emotional support.

Preface

HOW TO USE THIS BOOK

While the nursing aide competency evaluation program varies slightly from state to state, throughout the country the program measures the nursing assistant's knowledge and skills. All states require that you pass both a written and manual skills evaluation. The number of questions included on the written exam is different in various states. However, only multiple choice questions are asked. Which manual skills will be evaluated also varies from state to state. But all of the skills included are performed in your work as a nursing assistant.

This review book will assist you in preparing for both parts of the competency evaluation. Part Two deals with the written exam. Part Three reviews the skills tested in the manual evaluation. Basic nursing content areas are reviewed in Part Two. Each content area includes the key terms, an overview of the topic and general guidelines. The skills appropriate to each content area will be listed. Checklists describing how to perform these skills are included in Part Three. Review questions follow each topic area. After you have reviewed a topic, answer the test questions. You can either circle the answer with a pencil or write your answers on paper. Check your answers in Part Two, Section Two. Each answer includes the rationale as to why an answer is correct or incorrect. After each content area you will see (TNA 0000; LTCA 0000). This refers to the page numbers in *Mosby's Textbook for Nursing Assistants* 4th edition (TNA) and *Mosby's Textbook for Long-Term Care Assistants* 2nd edition (LTCA). The page numbers are provided to show where you can obtain more information about a content area. Page numbers are also found after the procedure titles in Part Three. The textbooks and page numbers can also be used if you need to review a topic more thoroughly. They can also be used if you do not totally understand an answer. You may find that you have answered some questions incorrectly. If so, you will need to review the topic more thoroughly. Study the specified pages in the textbook and test yourself again. You will probably answer the question correctly the second time. Keep reviewing and answering the questions until you are comfortable with the material. You can call Mosby–Year Book at 1-800-667-2968, if you need to purchase one of the textbooks. Ask to speak with "Customer Service." Someone will be happy to help you place an order. You can also buy a book at many community college bookstores. Or ask a local bookstore to place an order for you.

Sheila A. Sorrentino
CherylAnn S. Owoc

Contents

NURSING ASSISTANT
REVIEW
FOR COMPETENCY EVALUATION

PART ONE   OBRA and the Competency Evaluation Test

Nursing assistants, like other members of the health care team, must pass state licensing tests before practicing their profession. The test taken by nursing assistants consists of two parts—a written test and a manual skills test. This book can help you prepare for both parts of this test. Part One provides you with background information and helpful advice about the test. It also gives helpful advice about studying for and taking the tests. Part Two reviews important nursing content areas. Test questions will follow each content area. The correct answers are found in the back of that section. Reasons why an answer is correct or incorrect are included. Basic nursing procedures are presented in Part Three.

OMNIBUS BUDGET RECONCILIATION ACT OF 1987

In 1987 the US Congress passed the Omnibus Budget Reconciliation Act. Commonly referred to as "OBRA," this federal law applies to all 50 states. One purpose of this law is to improve the quality of care given in long-term care facilities. The passage of OBRA requires that all long-term care nursing assistants successfully complete a federally mandated and state approved nurse aide training program and pass a competency evaluation program in order to work as nursing assistants. While the basic requirements are the same in each state, some states have additional requirements. For example, OBRA requires 75 hours of training. Illinois, however, requires 120 hours of training. You need to know the requirements for the state in which you are working. Your instructor or supervisor can help provide you with this information. The state health department of licensing is another resource.

Each state is also required to maintain a registry for nursing assistants. This is a list of those nursing assistants who have successfully completed a training program and passed both parts of the state competency evaluation. Once placed on the registry, you will be required to renew your registry certificate at certain state-required time intervals. You will have to meet criteria determined by the state in order to keep your certificate current. One requirement is that you work in a long-term care facility for a required number of days. In addition, you will need to meet a required number of continuing education hours. Your current employer will be able to verify this information for you. This enables you to change employers without having to repeat the training program and the competency evaluation.

COMPETENCY EVALUATION

The nurse aide competency evaluation consists of two parts. There is a written test and a manual skills evaluation. The written test consists of multiple-choice questions. The number of questions will vary from state to state. For example, one state may have a test with 75 questions. Another state's test may ask 85 questions. Each question or statement will have four possible answers. Only one answer is correct. (How to take multiple choice tests is discussed on pp. 7 and 8.) You will be given enough time to complete the test. Usually there is about 1 minute to read and answer each question. Some questions will take less than a minute to read and answer. Other questions will take longer. You should have enough time to take the test without feeling rushed or hurried.

The skills evaluation involves demonstrating selected skills that you learned in your training program. This part of the competency examination is discussed in Part Three.

REGISTERING FOR THE COMPETENCY EVALUATION

A completed application and the appropriate fees must be sent to the testing agency by your sponsor. This is usually the person who gave you the application and a copy of the candidate handbook. It may be someone at the facility where you work or where you took your training course. Once the application and fees are received, you are notified of your evaluation date and location. All evaluation centers are handicapped accessible. However, if you need any special accommodations, you should notify your sponsor immediately.

Fees for the Nurse Aide Competency Evaluation have been established and may vary from state to state. There are fees for:

a. The first administration of both the Written Evaluation and the Manual Skills Evaluation
b. Retaking the Written Evaluation
c. Retaking the Manual Skills Evaluation
d. A surcharge for an oral administration of the Written Evaluation
e. Replacement of a lost Manual Skills Evaluation Admission Ticket
f. Non-cancellation of the Manual Skills Evaluation
g. Rescheduling of the Written Evaluation
h. Hand-scored verification of electronic scoring
 i. Duplicate evaluation results

You will be eligible to be placed on the Nursing Assistant Registry once you have passed both the Written and the Manual Skills Evaluations. When you receive notification that you have passed both evaluations, your sponsor will assist you in applying for the Registry. Fees for the registry may include:

a. Placement on the registry
b. Registry renewal

c. Updating the registry record (usually includes a new certificate)

d. Registration for out-of-state candidates

Fees are either paid by you, the facility where you work, or the institution where you received your nursing assistant aide training. Your sponsor will be able to tell you who is responsible for paying. If you need to pay the fees, you may need to purchase a money order. The money order must display your name. Personal checks may not be accepted.

PREPARING FOR THE COMPETENCY EVALUATION

Almost everyone dreads taking tests. Even taking a driver's license test causes fear and anxiety in most individuals. Professionals such as doctors, nurses, lawyers, accountants, and teachers experience anxiety about their licensing examinations as well. These feelings occur even though they have studied for many years. When it comes to taking tests, people often think one or more of the following:

"What if I don't pass?"

"I don't know enough."

"I don't do well on tests."

"I was never a good student."

"What if I forgot everything?"

"I wish I would have studied harder."

These thoughts and feelings are all very normal. If used wisely, anxiety can actually help you do well. When you are anxious, that means you are concerned. Being concerned usually results in some action. You can continue to worry, which only causes more anxiety. And more anxiety results in even greater worry. Or you can study and prepare for the test. That will help increase your confidence as you recall or clarify what you have learned. Anxiety will decrease as confidence increases.

STUDYING FOR AN EXAM

Developing good study skills

1. Spend as much time as needed each week reviewing the answers to the workbook and any other assignments. (A rough guide is to study 2 hours for every hour spent in class.)

2. Read each workbook and worksheet question carefully and isolate the "action" words that tell you what information is needed for your answer. Some examples of "action" words are: explain, list, identify, and define. Highlight these words by circling or underlining them. Then be certain that you do exactly what is required by these "action" words.

3. Underline important information in the questions that will have a bearing on your answer. For example: What are infections that are acquired while an individual is in the hospital called?

4. Jot brief notes to yourself as you read each workbook and worksheet question. This will enable you to retain these ideas.

5. Review the educational objectives and outline the study material to remind yourself of the key ideas and their relationships. In addition, read through the introductions, the key terms and concepts, and answer any review questions.

6. Identify any areas that are unclear and strengthen your understanding of these "weak" areas by restudying them.
7. Gain insights or study tips by studying with a partner or a study group.

Organizing class notes

1. Read through your notes. Make certain you understand them. Fill in any important missing notes. Make any additional notations (in a different color) alongside the original notes or on the back of the previous page.
2. Using a contrasting color, underline the key words and definitions and topic headings to recall words and the principal points of the topic.
3. Anticipate exam questions. Make up questions and practice writing answers. Check them for accuracy and completeness. Reread and rewrite these answers until you can give quick, complete responses.
4. Make index cards for hard to remember facts or to use as quiz cards (i.e., abbreviations).
5. Prepare study sheets for complex information. Select the information to be studied. Briefly outline it with all the information and facts about that topic on this sheet. Read through these sheets several times.
6. Multisensory learning helps you to remember more. Use as many of the senses as you can. Tape your notes and listen to them just before bed; review them again in the morning.
7. Use any memory devices that work for you.

STUDYING FOR THE COMPETENCY EVALUATION

Preparation for the competency evaluation began the first day of your nursing assistant course. The program included the basic nursing content areas and skills that you needed to know to provide safe, quality care. Reviewing your textbook and class notes is an important step in preparing for the competency evaluation. It will help you with both the written and manual portions.

The following suggestions can help you prepare for the competency evaluation and decrease your anxiety.

1. You should begin studying 2 to 3 weeks before the exam. Plan to study for 1 to 2 hours each day.
2. Decide on a specific time to study. This should be when you will not have many interruptions. It may be early in the morning before other family members are awake. You may want to study when family members have left for work or school. Some people like to study after everyone has gone to bed. You will need to choose a study time that is best for you.
3. Pick a specific place to study. This area should be quiet, well-lighted, and comfortable. You should have enough room to write and to spread out your books.
4. While you want to study in a quiet area, do not try to make this area absolutely noise free. Remember that the testing area will not be absolutely quiet. You want to be able to concentrate and not be distracted by the noise and movements around you.
5. Collect everything you need before settling down to study. This includes your nursing assistant textbook, your review book, notes from your training program, pencils, pens, or writing paper.

6. Take short breaks when you need them. Take a break when your mind begins to wander or if you feel sleepy.
7. Develop a study plan. Study one content area before going on to the next. For example, study personal hygiene before moving on to vital signs. Do not jump from one subject to another. Do not study oral hygiene, then blood pressure measurement, and then bathing.
8. Use a variety of ways to study. For example, you can use index cards to help you review abbreviations and terminology. Put the abbreviation or term on the front of the card and place the meaning on the back. You can take the cards with you and review them whenever you have a break. Taping key points is another study technique. You can listen to the tape while cooking, doing dishes, or riding in the car. Study groups are another way to help prepare for the exam. Other learners from your class may be taking the exam, too. By forming a study group, you can quiz each other. There are many ways to study. Find the ways that work best for you.
9. Remember that you passed your nursing assistant training program. That means you have passed many tests given by your instructor. You have already been successful taking tests! You have the knowledge and skills of a nursing assistant.

TAKING THE COMPETENCY EVALUATION

The written and manual skills examinations are usually taken on different days unless special arrangements are made. Your instructor or supervisor will assist you in determining where to take the tests and how to complete the required application form. The fee for the competency evaluation must be sent with your application.

Once your application has been processed, you will be notified about the date and time of your tests. Your admission tickets will be mailed to the address on your application form. You need to take your admission ticket with you to each part of the examination. Notify your instructor or supervisor if you have not received your admission ticket a week before your test date. If you need to change the date of your examination, notify your instructor or supervisor as soon as possible. In addition to your admission ticket, you may need to take a government-issued photo identification (driver's license) with you to the testing center for both the written and manual examinations.

You must arrive on time. Otherwise you will not be allowed to take the tests. Make sure you know the exact location of the test site and room. Actually drive or take transportation to the test site a few days or a week in advance. Making a "dry run" will let you know how much travel time you need and exactly where you are going.

Remember, you have already passed a nursing assistant course! Be positive and confident! But also remember that your physical comfort and mental well-being are important when taking the competency evaluation. The following suggestions can help you prepare both physically and mentally:

- Get a good night's sleep. Go to bed early enough so that you will not oversleep or be too tired to get up. You will not be able to think clearly if you are tired. Make sure your alarm clock is properly set.
- Do not "cram" the evening before or the day of the test. Last minute cramming only increases your anxiety. Do something relaxing with family

and friends. Many people find exercise to be helpful before a test. Walking, jogging, aerobics, swimming, and bicycling have both physical and mental benefits.

- Do deep breathing and muscle relaxation exercises when you feel tense or anxious.
- Eat only familiar foods the day before and the day of the exam. Do not eat foods that could cause stomach or intestinal upset.
- Avoid drinking large amounts of coffee, colas, water, or other beverages. You do not want to have to leave the test center to use the restroom. Nor do you want to be uncomfortable with a full bladder.
- Do not skip breakfast. Eat a nourishing meal before the test. Good nutrition helps you to think clearly.
- Wear comfortable clothes. You may want to dress in layers so that you are prepared for a cold or warm room. Extra clothes can be taken off if the room is too warm.
- If you are a woman, remember that worry and anxiety can affect your menstrual cycle. Wear a panty liner, sanitary napkin, or tampon if you think your period may start. This will eliminate worry about soiling your clothing during the test.
- Bring required information with you. You may be asked to bring a government issued photo identification (such as your driver's license) or a Substitute for Photo ID Form and an admission card. The admission card is sent to you by the testing agency. If you have not received your Admission Ticket by the Monday before your requested evaluation date, or if you have lost it, you need to notify your sponsor immediately.
- Take several sharpened number 2 pencils with erasers. Evaluation centers may not supply pencils.
- Do not take books, notes, papers, other reference materials, or calculators with you. These will not be allowed in the testing room.
- Allow plenty of time for travel, traffic, and parking.
- Arrive at your assigned Written Evaluation Center at least 30 minutes before the evaluation is to begin. Most centers will **NOT** admit you if you are late.
- Arrive early enough to use the restroom before the test begins.
- Do not talk about the test with others. Their panic or anxiety may affect your self confidence.
- No evaluation materials or notes are allowed to be taken out of the testing room.
- Listen carefully and follow all instructions given by the proctor (the person administering the test). Be sure and read all directions very carefully. Once the test has begun, you will not be allowed to ask any questions.
- You will not be allowed to ask questions about the content of the test questions (for example, "What does this word mean?" or "What do they mean by this question?").
- Cheating of any kind will not be allowed. If the proctor sees you giving or receiving any type of assistance, your test booklet will be taken and you will be asked to leave the testing site.

When you receive the exam, make certain you have all the test pages. Read and follow all directions carefully. If a computer answer sheet is being used, make certain that you fill the bubble completely. If you make a mistake, erase the wrong answer completely. Do not make any stray marks on the paper. Not erasing completely or leaving stray marks could cause the computer to misinterpret your answer.

Pace yourself during the examination. Do not spend time on difficult questions. First, answer all of the questions that you know. Then go back and answer the difficult ones. Answer all questions by eliminating and narrowing your choices. Always read the question or statement carefully and identify the key words. Know which words can make a statement correct (i.e., may, can, usually, most, at least, sometimes). The use of the word "except" can make a question a false statement.

ANSWERING MULTIPLE-CHOICE QUESTIONS

The written exam will consist of only multiple-choice questions. Each question will have four answer choices. Only one answer will be correct. Although some questions may appear to have more than one possible answer, there is only *one best answer.*

The following guidelines will help you answer multiple-choice questions:

- Always read the question or statement carefully. Do *not* scan or glance at a question. Scanning or glancing can cause you to miss important key words. Read each word of the question.
- Before reading the answers, decide what the answer is in your own words. Then read each answer carefully. Select the *one best answer.* Choose your answer after you have read all four choices.
- **DO NOT READ INTO A QUESTION.** Take the question as it is asked. Do not add your own thoughts and ideas to the question. Do not assume or suppose "what if." Just respond to the information provided.
- Trust your common sense. If you are unsure of an answer, select your first choice. **DO NOT CHANGE** your answer unless you are **ABSOLUTELY** sure of the correct answer. Your first reaction is probably the best. Studies have proven that the first reaction is usually correct. Do not change the answer unless you are positive that your first choice was wrong.
- Look for the key words in every question. Sometimes key words will be highlighted, underlined, or in italics. Common key words include: always, never, first, except, best, not, correct, incorrect, true, or false.
- Be careful of answers with the following key words or phrases: always, never, every, only, all, none, at all times, or at no time. These words and phrases do not allow for exceptions. In nursing, exceptions are generally present. However, sometimes answers containing those words are correct. For example, which of the following are correct and which are incorrect:
  a. Always use a turning sheet.
  b. Never shake linens.
  c. Never place linen on the floor.
  d. The cotton drawsheet must always cover the plastic drawsheet.
  e. The signal light must always be attached to the bed.
  f. Soap is used for all baths.
  The correct answers are b, c, and d. Incorrect answers are a, e, and f.
- Omit those answers that are obviously wrong. Then choose the best of the remaining answers.

- Pace yourself during the exam. Do not spend time on difficult questions. First, answer all of the questions that you know. Then go back and answer the difficult ones. Sometimes you will remember the answer later. Or another test question may give you a clue to the one you skipped. Spending too much time on a question can cost you valuable time later.

- Go back to the questions you skipped. Answer all questions by eliminating and narrowing your choices. Be sure to mark an answer even if you are not sure. The question will definitely be counted wrong if you do not choose an answer.

- Review the test a second time before turning it in for completeness and accuracy.

- Make sure you have answered each question. Also verify that you have only given one answer for each question.

- Remember that the test has not been designed to trick or confuse you. The written competency evaluation tests what you know, not what you do not know. You know more than you will be asked.

- Multiple choice tests do not require total recall. The answer has been provided. You only have to select the *one best* answer from the four choices.

- Avoid last minute cramming. Not only will it increase your stress level, but it will cause you to confuse facts and information.

PART TWO   The Written Evaluation

Section I   Review and Sample Questions

NOTE: The authors believe that every patient and resident should be viewed as a unique *person*. *Person* is used in the text when referring to the patient and resident. However, the competency evaluation is intended for nursing assistants working in long-term care facilities. Test questions may contain the word "resident." Therefore, *resident* is used in the review questions so you can apply your learning to the long-term care setting.

Chapter 1   *The nursing assistant*

WORDS TO REMEMBER

assault Intentionally attempting or threatening to touch a person's body without the person's consent

battery Unauthorized touching of a person's body without the person's consent

civil laws Laws concerned with relationships between people; private law

crime An act that is a violation of a criminal law

criminal law Laws concerned with offenses against the public and society in general; public law

defamation Injuring a person's name and reputation by making false statements to a third person

empathy The ability to see things from another person's point of view

ethics Knowledge of what is right and wrong conduct

false imprisonment Unlawful restraint or restriction of a person's movement

fraud Saying or doing something to trick, fool, or deceive another person

invasion of privacy A violation of a person's right not to have his or her name, photograph, or private affairs exposed or made public without giving consent

legal That which pertains to law

libel Defamation through written statements

malpractice Negligence by a professional person

negligence An unintentional wrong in which a person fails to act in a reasonable and careful manner and causes harm to a person or to the person's property

slander Defamation through oral statements

tort A wrong committed against a person or the person's property

NURSING ASSISTANTS IN LONG-TERM CARE

The nursing assistant in long-term care facilities performs simple and basic nursing functions under the supervision of a nurse. The RN and/or LPN is responsible for assigning and supervising your work. You do not make decisions about what should or should not be done for a person. If you do not understand the directions or instructions, ask the nurse for clarification before giving care. Perform no function or task that you have not been taught how to do or that you do not feel prepared to perform.

You give care relating to the personal hygiene, safety, nutrition, exercise, and elimination needs. There are certain functions, procedures, and tasks that you should **NEVER** do. You must understand what you can and cannot do as a nursing assistant:

• Never give medications of any kind. This includes medications given orally, rectally, by injection, or directly into the bloodstream through an intravenous line. Both prescription (those ordered by a doctor) and over-the-counter (such as aspirin and vitamins) medications are included.

- Never insert tubes or objects into a body opening or remove them from the body. Exceptions to this rule would be enemas, thermometers, or rectal tubes once you have been taught these skills and been supervised performing them.
- Never take oral or telephone orders from doctors. If you answer the telephone or a doctor wants to give you an order, ask the doctor to wait and promptly find an RN or LPN to speak with the doctor.
- Never perform procedures that require sterile technique. Sterile technique and procedures require skills, knowledge, and judgment beyond the training nursing assistants receive. You may assist the RN or LPN during a sterile procedure, but you may not perform the procedure yourself.
- Never tell the person or family the person's diagnosis or medical or surgical treatment plans. The doctor is responsible for informing the person or family about the diagnosis and treatment. Nurses may further clarify what the doctor has told the person and the family.
- Never discuss the person or the person's treatment with anyone except the RN and/or LPN supervising your work. "Shop talk" is one of the most common causes of invasion of privacy.
- Never diagnose or prescribe treatments or medications for any person. Only doctors can diagnose and prescribe.
- Never supervise the work of other nursing assistants. RNs and LPNs are legally responsible for supervising the work of nursing assistants.
- Never ignore an order or request to do something that you cannot do or that is beyond the scope of practice as a nursing assistant. Promptly explain to the nurse why you cannot carry out the order or request. The nurse will assume you are doing what you were told to do unless you explain otherwise. The person's care cannot be neglected. (TNA 19; LTCA 14–15)

The desire to make the lives of the elderly and disabled persons happier, easier, and less painful is an essential characteristic for health team members in long-term care. In addition to wanting to help people to be as happy and independent as possible, it is important that you *believe* each person has value as a human being no matter how old, ill, or disabled that person may be. Certain traits, attitudes, and manners allow you to do your job well. These include dependability, consideration, cheerfulness, empathy, patience, trustworthiness, respectfulness, courtesy, conscientiousness, honesty, cooperation, and self-awareness. (TNA 30–31; LTCA 17–18)

As a health care worker, you serve as an example to others. It is important that you use good health and personal hygiene practices. You must look clean, neat, and professional. (TNA 18–24; LTCA 18–19)

As a member of both the nursing and health care teams, you work closely with the RNs, LPNs, and other nursing assistants. Your ability to work well with others will affect how well you function as a nursing assistant and the quality of care received by your residents. This will include planning and organizing your work to give safe, thorough care and prioritizing your time appropriately. (TNA 38–40; LTCA 23–24)

Take note!

- Understand the roles, functions, and responsibilities in your job description. Report to work on time. Call the facility, according to facility guidelines, if you cannot report to work.
- Act in an ethical and legal manner at all times. Follow your supervisor's directions and instructions. Ask for clarification when you do not understand your assignment.
- Report the person's or family's complaints and your observations to the nurse promptly. Measure, record, and report accurately.
- Do not use the telephones, supplies, or equipment of the person's or the facility for personal use. Do not waste supplies or abuse the equipment.
- Do not discuss your personal problems with any person or family.
- Discuss assignment priorities with the nurse.
- Estimate how much time is needed for each person, procedure, and task. Plan care around meals, visiting hours, therapies, and recreational or social activities.
- Identify when you will need help from a co-worker. Ask for assistance when needed. Tell the co-worker the approximate time you will need help.
- Schedule any equipment or rooms as needed. Review procedures and collect supplies beforehand.

Questions for review (Answers to these questions are on page 83)

Circle the best answer.
1. A nurse assigns you a task. You do not understand the instructions. You should
   a. try your best.
   b. ask the resident what to do.
   c. ask the nurse for clarification.
   d. refuse to carry out the request.
2. Nursing assistants
   a. never give medications.
   b. can supervise other nursing assistants.

c. do not perform personal hygiene measures.

d. must perform all tasks and procedures as directed by the nurse.

3. Who is responsible for telling the resident and family about diagnosis and treatment?
   a. The nurse
   b. The physician
   c. Any staff member
   d. The nursing assistant

4. Which is **not** a good quality or characteristic for a nursing assistant?
   a. Following orders and instructions carefully
   b. Trying to change a resident's beliefs or values
   c. Reporting care, observations, and measurements accurately
   d. Being aware of your own feelings, strengths, and weaknesses

5. You are planning and organizing your assignment. Which is **false?**
   a. Collect supplies as you need them.
   b. List necessary care or procedures on a schedule.
   c. Plan care around meals, visiting hours, therapies, and activities.
   d. Ask a co-worker for help when needed. Give the approximate time you will need assistance.

LEGAL CONSIDERATIONS

Legal considerations relate to laws. Torts (from a French word meaning *wrong*) are part of civil law. They may be intentional or unintentional. The following torts are common to health care:

Negligence is an unintentional wrong. The person did not mean or intend to cause harm. The negligent person failed to act in a reasonable and careful manner and, as a result, caused harm to the person or property of another. As a nursing assistant you are legally responsible (*liable*) for your own actions. A nurse may direct you to do something that is beyond the legal scope of your role. Or you may be asked to do something for which you have not been prepared. While the nurse will be held liable as your supervisor, you are in no way relieved of personal liability. **You are responsible for your own actions.**

Defamation (libel and slander), assault and battery, false imprisonment, invasion of privacy, and fraud are intentional torts. You can protect yourself from defamation by never making false statements about a co-worker or any other person.

Assault and battery may result in both civil and criminal charges. Consent is the important factor in assault and battery. The person must consent to any procedure, treatment, or other act that involves touching the body. The person has the right to withdraw consent at any time. You can protect yourself from assault by not attempting or threatening to touch the person, thereby having the person fear bodily harm. Explaining to the person what is to be done and getting the person's consent can protect you from being accused of battery. The consent may be verbal or nonverbal (a gesture).

False imprisonment is the unlawful restraint or restriction of a person's freedom of movement. Threat of restraint or actual physical restraint constitutes false imprisonment.

Invasion of privacy is another tort. You must treat persons with respect and ensure their privacy. (TNA 26-28; LTCA 21-23)

Take note!

- You are legally responsible for your own actions.
- What you do or do not do can lead to a lawsuit if harm results to the person or property of another.
- You can protect the persons you care for and yourself from negligent acts by using common sense. Ask yourself if what you are doing is safe for the person.
- The person must consent to any procedure, treatment, or other act that involves touching the body.
- Keep all resident information confidential.

Questions for review (Answers to these questions are on page 83)

Circle the best answer.

1. The intentional attempt or threat to touch a person's body without the person's consent is
   a. assault.
   b. battery.
   c. defamation.
   d. false imprisonment.

2. Which of the following would probably **NOT** be negligent conduct?
   a. A resident's dentures break after being dropped by the nursing assistant.
   b. A resident is burned because a nursing assistant applied a warm water bottle that was too hot.
   c. A nursing assistant reports a resident's complaint of chest pain and difficulty breathing. The resident has a heart attack and dies.
   d. The side rails have been ordered for a confused resident. The nursing assistant leaves the side rails down. The resident falls out of bed and breaks a hip.

3. A resident refuses to have a bath. The nursing assistant tells her that she is going to have a bath whether she likes it or not. This is an example of
   a. assault.
   b. battery.
   c. defamation.
   d. false imprisonment.

4. A nurse tells you to give Mr. Smith a sleeping pill. You tell the nurse that you are not allowed to give medications. She tells you to go ahead and not to worry because no one else will know. She also tells you she will accept the blame if anything goes wrong. Which statement is **TRUE**?
   a. You have to give the pill because the nurse directed you to do so.
   b. You have nothing to worry about. The nurse said she would take the blame.
   c. You are legally responsible for your own actions. Mr. Smith can sue you for causing harm.
   d. Mr. Smith cannot sue you. He can only sue the nurse because she is legally responsible for your actions.
5. These statements are about negligence. Which is **TRUE**?
   a. It is an intentional tort.
   b. Harm was caused to a person or a person's property.
   c. The negligent person acted in a reasonable manner.
   d. Nursing assistants cannot be held liable for any negligent acts.

RESIDENT RIGHTS

The Omnibus Budget Reconciliation Act of 1987 (OBRA) is concerned with the quality of life, health, and safety of residents. Some of the many OBRA requirements relate to resident rights and the quality of life.

Nursing facility residents have certain rights under federal and state laws. Residents have rights as citizens of the United States. They also have rights relating to their everyday lives and care in a nursing facility. Nursing facilities must protect and promote resident rights. Residents must be free to exercise their rights without facility interference. Legal representatives exercise the rights for those residents who are incompetent (not able).

Nursing facilities must inform residents of their rights. They must be informed orally and in writing. This information is given before or during admission to the facility. It must be given in the language used and understood by the resident.

OBRA requires that nursing facilities care for residents in a manner that promotes dignity, self-worth, and physical, psychological, and emotional well-being. Protecting resident rights is one way to promote quality of life. Personal choice, privacy, participation in group activities, having personal property, and freedom from restraint show respect for the person.

The resident is spoken to in a polite and courteous manner. Giving good, honest, and thoughtful care enhances the resident's quality of life. (TNA 140–143; LTCA 8–10)

OBRA and state laws require the reporting of elderly abuse. If abuse is suspected, it must be reported. When and how to report abuse varies in each state. If you need to report suspected abuse, you must give as much information as possible. The reporting agency will take action based on the information given. They act immediately if the situation is life-threatening. Sometimes the help of police or the courts is necessary. (TNA 145; LTCA 106)

A summary of Resident Rights is found in Part Three, "Skills Evaluation," on pages 108–110.

Questions for review (Answers to these questions are on page 84)

Circle the best answer.
1. The following statements are about resident rights. Which statement is **TRUE**?
   a. Residents' mail can be opened by any facility employee.
   b. Residents have the right to have telephone conversations in private.
   c. Residents' closets and drawers can be searched to look for lost items.
   d. Residents may only visit with others in an area where they can be seen and heard by others.
2. The following statements are about the care of residents. Which is **FALSE**?
   a. Residents must be free from abuse, neglect, and mistreatment.
   b. Residents can be restrained to prevent them from leaving the facility.
   c. Participation in activities is important for residents' quality of life.
   d. Allowing personal choice is important for residents' quality of life.
3. Under the Omnibus Budget Reconciliation Act (OBRA), a resident has all of the following rights except one. Which is **FALSE**?
   a. The right to be treated with respect
   b. The right to visit with others in private
   c. The right to have a private room in which to live
   d. The right to have an environment that is clean and safe
4. Who decides how the resident's hair should be styled?
   a. The nurse
   b. The family
   c. The resident
   d. The nursing assistant
5. Which of the following promote the resident's quality of life?
   a. Having John Smith's family take his favorite books home
   b. Insisting Bea Nice attend the Sing-Along in the dayroom

c. Helping Mr. Green get to the activities room in time for the bowling match

d. Dressing Mrs. Jones in a stained dress since she will only get food on it anyway

PRIVACY AND CONFIDENTIALITY

Every person has the right not to have his or her name, photograph, or private affairs exposed or made public without having given consent. A violation of this right is an *invasion of privacy*. You must treat every person with respect and ensure their privacy. Only health care workers involved in the person's care should see, handle, or examine the resident's body. The right to privacy must still be protected even after death. (TNA 28; LTCA 8–9)

Confidentiality in relation to the person's information and records is similar to the right to privacy. The person has the right to expect that information will be shared with other health care workers in a wise and careful manner. Only members of the health team involved with the person's care should see the person's record. You must recognize the confidential nature of the person's information. Some people are very sensitive about such things as their age or wearing a wig or dentures. (TNA 28; LTCA 8–9)

Providing for privacy and keeping medical and personal information confidential show respect for the individual. This also protects the person's dignity.

Take note!

- Make sure the person is covered when being moved in the corridors.
- Screen the person when giving care. Use privacy curtains or close the door.
- Expose only the body part involved in a treatment or procedure.
- Do not discuss the person or the person's treatment with anyone except the nurse supervising your work. "Shop talk" is one of the most common causes of invasion of privacy.
- Residents have the right to visit with others in private. They have the right to visit in an area where they cannot be seen or heard by others.
- Residents have the right to have telephone calls in private.
- Residents have the right to send and receive mail without interference. Letters sent and received by the resident must not be opened by others without the resident's permission.
- Do not go through a resident's closet, drawers, purse, or other space without the person's knowledge and consent.

Questions for review (Answers to these questions are on page 84)

Circle the best answer.

1. Which is an invasion of privacy?
   a. A resident is covered while being moved on a stretcher.
   b. The door to the resident's room is closed while a treatment is being given.
   c. A resident is being given a back rub. Only the resident's back is uncovered.
   d. The resident's condition and treatment are discussed with the resident's cousin who works in the dietary department.

2. Which will **NOT** protect the person's right to privacy?
   a. Asking visitors to leave the room when care must be given.
   b. Exposing only the body part involved in a treatment or procedure.
   c. Making sure the person is covered when being moved in corridors.
   d. Staying with the person while he or she uses the telephone or visits with others.

3. Which of the following individuals need to read the resident's chart?
   a. Physicians and nurses only
   b. Friends, family, and members of the health team
   c. Any member of the health team who is interested
   d. Members of the health team involved in the resident's care

4. The following statements are about resident rights to privacy. Which statement is **TRUE**?
   a. Residents' mail can be opened by any facility employee.
   b. Residents have the right to have telephone conversations in private.
   c. Residents' closets and drawers can be searched to look for lost items.
   d. Residents may only visit with others in an area where they can be seen and heard by others.

Chapter 2   *Communication*

WORDS TO REMEMBER

chart Another term for the medical record

communication The exchange of information; a message sent is received and interpreted by the intended person

Kardex A type of card file that summarizes information found in the medical record; includes medications, treatments, diagnosis, routine care measures, and special equipment used by the patient or resident

medical record A written account of a person's illness and response to the treatment and care given by the health team; chart

minimum data set (MDS) A form used by nurses in nursing facilities to assess a resident's mental, physical, and psychosocial functioning

nonverbal communication Communication that does not involve words

nursing care plan A written guide that gives direction about the nursing care a person should receive

nursing diagnosis A statement describing a health problem that can be treated by nursing measures

objective data Information that can be seen, heard, felt, or smelled by another person; signs

observation Using the senses of sight, hearing, touch, and smell to collect information about a person

recording Writing or charting a person's care and observations

reporting A verbal account of a person's care and observations

resident assessment protocol (RAP) Triggers and guidelines used in developing the comprehensive care plan

signs Objective data

subjective data That which is reported by a person and cannot be observed by using the senses; symptoms

symptoms Subjective data

triggers Clues that direct the caregiver to the appropriate resident assessment protocol (RAP)

verbal communication Communication that uses the written or spoken word

COMMUNICATION AMONG THE HEALTH CARE TEAM

Communication among health team members is important for coordinated and effective resident care. Information must be shared about what has been done and what needs to be done for a person. It must be given in a logical, concise, and orderly manner.

The person's record (chart) is a permanent written account of the person's condition and response to treatment. It is a legal document. The chart has various sections for easy use. Each page has the person's name, room number, and other identifying information. Each facility has policies about the type of forms used, who records information, and how it is to be recorded.

Usually all professional health workers involved in the person's care have access to the medical record. Some facilities do not let nursing assistants read charts. If not, the nurse shares necessary information with the nursing assistant.

Take note!

- When charting, use ink and write legibly. Make sure spelling, grammar, and punctuation are correct. Do not erase or use correction fluid. Use a line to cross out the incorrect part. Write "error" over it with your initials. Then record the new entry. Some facilities use "mistaken entry" rather than "error." Follow your facility's policy for correcting errors.
- Entries must be timed and dated. Sign all entries with your name and title. Never skip lines. Make sure each page is properly identified.
- Never chart a procedure or treatment until it is completed.
- Use the person's exact words whenever possible. Use quotation marks for exact quotes made by the person.
- Be accurate, concise, and factual. Avoid terms with more than one meaning. Record in a logical and sequential manner.
- Use the Kardex as a quick and easy source of the person's information and routines found in the medical record.
- Carry a note pad and pen with you. Make notes of your observations. (TNA 65–67; LTCA 32 –37)

Questions for review (Answers to these questions are on page 85)

Circle the best answer.

1. Communication is
   a. the exchange of information.
   b. a verbal account of resident care and observations.
   c. using sight, hearing, touch, and smell to collect information.
   d. a written account of the resident's illness and response to treatment.
2. The main purpose of the resident's record is to
   a. serve as evidence of resident care in court.
   b. communicate information about resident care.
   c. serve as a history of the resident's illness and treatment.
   d. provide the family with a written account of the resident's care and treatment.
3. Each page of the resident's record
   a. is the same.
   b. must be numbered.
   c. must be signed by the doctor.
   d. must have the resident's identifying information.
4. Who can read the resident's chart?
   a. The resident or family
   b. Any interested health worker
   c. The physician and nurses only
   d. Members of the health team involved in the resident's care
5. Which statement about charting is *incorrect?*
   a. All entries must be signed.
   b. All entries must be in pencil.
   c. No blank lines are left in an entry.
   d. All entries must be dated and signed.
6. The nursing care plan
   a. is also called the Kardex.
   b. is written by the physician.
   c. is the same for all residents.
   d. consists of actions nursing personnel should take to help a resident.
7. A resident has a stabbing pain in his chest. This is an example of
   a. objective data.
   b. collective data.
   c. subjective data.
   d. comprehensive data.
8. The quickest way to find out how many times a day Mr. Adams is to walk in the hall would be to
   a. ask the physician.
   b. check the Kardex.
   c. look in the nurses' notes.
   d. look in the physical therapy report.
9. In charting, you should *not*
   a. erase errors.
   b. sign each entry.
   c. use the resident's exact words.
   d. chart each treatment after it is completed.
10. You are required to report to the nurse about the resident's care and condition. This report is made
    a. at the beginning of the shift.
    b. at the end of the shift.
    c. at the midpoint of the shift.
    d. whenever the resident's condition requires it or as requested by the nurse.

THE HEARING IMPAIRED PERSON

Hearing loss is a common problem of aging. The impairment is often a gradual process. Many people deny that they have difficulty hearing. They may not be aware of the problem. Speaking too loudly, leaning forward to hear, and turning and cupping the better ear toward the speaker are all signs of impaired hearing. Answering questions or responding inappropriately and asking for words to be repeated are other signs of hearing impairment. To prevent embarrassment, the hearing impaired person may avoid social situations. Loneliness, boredom, and the feelings of being left out often result.

Hearing impaired persons may wear hearing aids, read lips, or use sign language. Some will develop speech problems, making it difficult to understand them.

A hearing aid is an instrument that makes sound louder. This includes background noises as well as speech. These devices are expensive and must be handled with care. Only removable earpieces can be washed. This is done daily. Batteries need to be checked and replaced at regular intervals. (TNA 584–587; LTCA 499–500)

Take note!

- Gain the attention of the hearing impaired person as you approach. Do not startle him or her. Lightly touch the person's arm to alert the person of your presence.
- Face the person directly when speaking so your lips and expression can be seen. Stand in a good light, without shadows or glare. Speak clearly, distinctly, and slowly. Use a normal tone of voice. Do not shout. Do not chew gum, eat, or cover your mouth while speaking.
- State the topic of conversation first. Use short sentences and simple words. Write out important words or names. Repeat or rephrase statements when necessary. Be patient.
- Reduce or eliminate background noise.
- Be alert to messages being sent by your facial expressions, gestures, and body language. Give the person your full attention.
- If a hearing aid does not seem to work, check the following: battery placement, battery power, on-off switch, earpiece placement, and cleanliness of earpiece.

Questions for Review (Answers to these questions are on page 86)

Circle the best answer.

1. Which of the following is **NOT** a sign of hearing loss?
   a. Speaking too loudly
   b. Loneliness and boredom
   c. Asking for things to be repeated
   d. Answering questions inappropriately
2. A hearing aid
   a. makes sound louder.
   b. makes speech clearer.
   c. corrects hearing problems.
   d. eliminates background noise.
3. When communicating with a hearing impaired resident do **NOT**
   a. speak loudly.
   b. speak slowly.
   c. face the resident.
   d. speak in a normal tone of voice.
4. When cleaning a hearing aid with a removable earpiece, you should
   a. soak the earpiece in alcohol.
   b. wash the earpiece in soap and water.
   c. soak the entire hearing aid in hot water.
   d. scrub the earpiece vigorously to remove earwax.
5. You are talking to a hearing impaired resident. Which of the following actions is **FALSE**?
   a. State the topic of discussion.
   b. Write out important names and words.

   c. Use short sentences and simple words.
   d. Cover your mouth, smoke, or chew gum while talking.

MEDICAL TERMINOLOGY

Tables 1, 2, and 3 list the prefixes, roots, and suffixes of words commonly used in medical terminology. Table 4 lists common abbreviations. These tables are intended for quick review only. (TNA 739–745; LTCA 568–572)

Questions for review (Answers to these questions are on page 86)

Circle the best answer.

1. Paralysis on one side of the body is called
   a. hemiplegia.
   b. paraplegia.
   c. hemaplegia.
   d. quadriplegia.
2. The medical abbreviation for "before meals" is
   a. ac.
   b. pc.
   c. BM.
   d. NPO.
3. The medical abbreviation "prn" means
   a. as desired.
   b. immediately.
   c. when necessary.
   d. patient really needs.
4. The medical abbreviation for "twice a day" is
   a. qd.
   b. bid.
   c. tid.
   d. qid.
5. The physician has ordered that Mrs. Jones is "to go to physical therapy qod." That means that she will go
   a. every day.
   b. every other day.
   c. four times a day.
   d. every 4 hours.

Table 1

PREFIX	MEANING	EXAMPLE
a-, an-	without or not	anuria
ab-	away from	abduction
ad-	toward	adduction
bi-	double, two	bilateral
brady-	slow	bradycardia
dys-	bad, difficult, abnormal	dyspnea
hyper-	excessive, too much, high	hypertension
hypo-	under, decreased, less	hypothyroid
olig-	small, scanty	oliguria
poly-	many, much	polyuria
tachy-	fast, rapid	tachycardia

Table 2

ROOT	MEANING
abdomin(o)	abdomen
arterio	artery
arthr(o)	joint
broncho	bronchus, bronchi
card, cardi(o)	heart
cephal(o)	head
colo	colon, large intestine
crani(o)	skull
cyan(o)	blue
cyst(o)	bladder, cyst
derma	skin
encephal(o)	brain
enter(o)	intestines
gastr(o)	stomach
gluc(o)	sweetness, glucose
glyc(o)	sugar
hem, hema, hemo, hemat(o)	blood
hepat(o)	liver
hydr(o)	water
lith(o)	stone
my(o)	muscle
nephr(o)	kidney
neur(o)	nerve
ocul(o), ophthalm(o)	eye
oste(o)	bone
ot(o)	ear
phleb(o)	vein
pnea	breathing
psych(o)	mind
pulmo	lung
thromb(o)	clot, thrombus
urin(o)	urine
uro	urine, urinary tract, urination

Table 3

SUFFIX	MEANING	EXAMPLE
-algia	pain	cephalgia
-asis	condition, usually abnormal	metastasis
-emia	blood condition	anemia
-itis	inflammation	appendicitis
-oma	tumor	lipoma
-pathy	disease	neuropathy
-phasia	speaking	aphasia
-plegia	paralysis	hemiplegia
-stomy, ostomy	creation of an opening	colostomy
-uria	condition of the urine	hematuria

Table 4

ABBREVIATION	MEANING
abd	abdomen
ac	before meals
ADL	activities of daily living
ad lib	as desired
amb	ambulatory
bid	twice daily
BM	bowel movement
BP	blood pressure
BRP	bathroom privileges
c̄	with
CBR	complete bed rest
CVA	cerebrovascular accident, stroke
dc, d/c	discontinue
drsg	dressing
FBS	fasting blood sugar
FF	force fluids
h, hr	hour
H₂O	water
HS, hs	hour of sleep, bedtime
I&O	intake and output
IV	intravenous
ml	milliliter
NPO	nothing by mouth
O₂	oxygen
OOB	out of bed
OT	occupational therapy
pc	after meals
po, per os	by mouth
prn	when necessary
PT	physical therapy
q	every
qd	every day
qh	every hour
q2h, q3h	every two hours, every three hours
qhs	every night at bedtime
qid	four times a day
qod	every other day
ROM	range of motion
stat	immediately, at once
tid	three times a day
TPR	temperature, pulse and respiration
U/a, U/A, ua, u/a	urinalysis
VS, vs	vital signs
w/c	wheelchair
wt	weight

Chapter 3 — Understanding the persons you care for

WORDS TO REMEMBER

culture The values, beliefs, habits, likes, dislikes, customs, and characteristics of a group that are passed from one generation to the next

esteem The worth, value, or opinion one has of a person

impotence The inability of the male to have an erection

menopause The time when menstruation stops; it marks the end of the woman's reproductive years

religion Spiritual beliefs, needs, and practices

rigor mortis The stiffness or rigidity (*rigor*) of skeletal muscles that occurs after death (*mortis*)

self-actualization Experiencing one's potential

sex The physical activities involving the organs of reproduction; the activities are done for pleasure or to produce children

sexuality That which relates to one's sex; those physical, psychological, social, cultural, and spiritual factors that affect a person's feelings and attitudes about his or her sex

terminal illness An illness or injury for which there is no reasonable expectation of recovery

BASIC NEEDS

A need is defined as that which is necessary or desirable for maintaining life and mental well-being. Abraham Maslow identified five basic needs that must be met if a person is to survive and function. Lower level needs must be met before the higher level needs. People normally meet their own needs every day. Disease, illness, or disability can interfere with a person's attempt to meet these needs.

Physiological needs are the most important for survival. These are the needs for oxygen, food, water, elimination, and rest. Before moving on to higher needs, physical needs must be met.

Safety and security needs relate to the need for shelter, clothing, and protection from harm or danger. Many elderly people feel a loss of security and safety when admitted to a long-term care facility. They are moved from familiar, secure surroundings (home) to a strange place. Some become frightened, confused, or depressed. When admitting a person to a long-term care facility, you must function competently and efficiently. You need to convey courtesy, respect, and caring to the person and family. A person feels safer and more secure if he or she receives explanations about procedures first. Knowing how a procedure is to be done and what sensations or feelings to expect help the person cope.

The need for love and belonging relates to closeness, affection, belonging, love, and meaningful relationships with others. These needs are usually met by family and friends. If none exist, health care workers must meet these needs.

The need for esteem means the worth, value, or opinion one has of a person or oneself, seeing oneself as useful, and being well thought of by others. The elderly, disabled, or chronically ill often lack self-esteem. You can help the person feel worthwhile. Focus on the person's abilities and strengths and encourage independence.

The need for self-actualization means experiencing one's potential. It involves learning, understanding, and creating to the limit of one's capacity. This is the highest need and one that is rarely met completely. (TNA 75–77; LTCA 50–52)

Take note!

- Remember that each person is unique. Treat each individual as a person who can think, act, and make decisions.
- Help persons regain their sense of security. Be kind, understanding, and patient. Show them their surroundings, listen to their concerns, and explain all routines and procedures.
- Improve the quality of life for each person. Help each one regain as much physical and mental function as possible.
- Family and friends are important to the resident. They can help meet the basic needs and influence recovery. Treat them with respect and courtesy.

Questions for review (Answers to these questions are on page 86)

Circle the best answer.

1. To care effectively for residents, you must consider the whole person. What does this mean?
   a. The person's entire body must be considered intact.
   b. How the resident views himself or herself is important.
   c. Residents must be called by name, not their room and bed numbers.
   d. Residents must be viewed as having physical, psychological, social, and spiritual parts.
2. Mr. Michaels is a new resident. He says that he sees strange shadows and hears funny noises at night. Which basic need is affected?
   a. Physical
   b. Safety and security
   c. Love and belonging
   d. Esteem
3. Mrs. Smith says she feels "absolutely worthless" since confined to a wheelchair. She is a former nurse and has three children. Which basic need is affected?
   a. Physical
   b. Safety and security
   c. Love and belonging
   d. Esteem
4. Mrs. Hopkins is 97 years old. She has no living family members. Most of her friends have died. Two close friends are in other long-term care facilities. A lady from her church visits her during the holidays. Which basic need is affected?
   a. Physical
   b. Safety and security
   c. Love and belonging
   d. Esteem
5. Mrs. Adams asks for knitting supplies. She wants to make a sweater for her new granddaughter. Which basic need is involved?
   a. Physical
   b. Safety and security
   c. Love and belonging
   d. Self-actualization

CULTURE AND RELIGION

Culture influences health beliefs and practices and a person's behavior. You will care for people from different cultural backgrounds. These people may have family practices, food preferences, hygiene habits, and clothing styles that are different from your own. Some may speak and understand another language. Some cultural groups have beliefs about the causes and cures of illnesses.

Many persons find their religion to be a source of comfort and strength during illness or periods of loneliness. They may wish to observe certain religious practices and may appreciate a visit from their spiritual leader. (TNA 77; LTCA 52)

Take note!

- If a person requests a visit from their spiritual leader, be sure to promptly report that request to the nurse.
- Make sure the person's room is neat and orderly and that there is a chair available for the spiritual leader.
- Allow the person and spiritual leader privacy during the visit.
- Most Americans are of the Protestant, Roman Catholic, or Jewish faith.
- Individuals may not follow every belief and practice of their culture or religion.
- Remember that each person is unique. Do not judge the person by your own standards.

Questions for review (Answers to these questions are on page 86)

Circle the best answer.

1. Mrs. Greene refuses to eat certain foods because of her religious beliefs. The nursing assistant should
   a. tell the doctor.
   b. respect her religious beliefs and notify the nurse.
   c. tell Mrs. Greene that she will not receive anything else to eat.
   d. tell Mrs. Greene that she should eat the food because the doctor wants her to.
2. Mr. O'Malley tells you what it was like growing up in Ireland. The nursing assistant should
   a. change the subject.
   b. talk about his or her family.
   c. report it to the nurse immediately.
   d. listen to what Mr. O'Malley has to say.
3. Learning as much as you can about the resident's cultural beliefs is
   a. not important.
   b. not allowed in the health care facility.
   c. only important if the resident has no family or friends.
   d. important in providing care that will meet the resident's needs.
4. Mrs. Johnson is a Roman Catholic. She asks you to call a priest for her. You are a Protestant. You should

a. call your minister.
b. call the chaplain of the facility.
c. report the request to the nurse.
d. call the priest from the nearest parish.
5. Which statement is **FALSE**?
   a. Dietary practices may be influenced by both culture and religion.
   b. A person's cultural background probably influences health and illness practices.
   c. A person's religious and cultural practices are not allowed in the health care facility.
   d. A person may not follow all of the beliefs and practices of his or her religion or culture.

SOCIAL FUNCTIONING

Social relationships change throughout life. Most elderly people adjust to these changes. However, some experience loneliness. Separation from children, lack of companionship with friends, and death of a spouse are common causes of loneliness in the elderly.

For others, the roles of parent and child are reversed. Instead of the parent caring for the child, adult children care for elderly parents. The older person may feel a loss of dignity and self-respect. Tension can develop between them.

Retirement can be difficult. For some, the satisfaction and sense of pride that result from working are replaced with social emptiness and feelings of uselessness. Retirement often means reduced income. Severe financial difficulty may result.

No amount of preparation is ever enough for the emptiness and changes that result when death takes a spouse. The individual loses more than a husband or wife. A friend, lover, companion, and confidant are also gone. The grief felt by the surviving spouse may be very great. Serious physical and mental health problems can result. (TNA 135; LTCA 99)

Other family members and friends can be very supportive of the elderly person. The person should be allowed to visit in private and without unnecessary interruptions. Treat visitors with courtesy and respect. They may be very concerned and frightened about the person's condition and care. Refer any questions they may have about the person to the nurse. (TNA 134–135; LTCA 96)

Take note!

- Encourage participation in social activities. Talk about subjects that interest the person. Provide newspapers, magazines, and television for persons able to enjoy them.
- Know the visiting policies of your facility. Also know the special considerations that may be allowed for a person.
- A person may become upset or tired from visitors. Report your observations to the nurse.

Questions for review (Answers to these questions are on page 87)

Circle the best answer.
1. Aging is
   a. a normal process.
   b. the result of injury.
   c. a disease process.
   d. the result of illness.
2. Retirement may result in
   a. lowered income.
   b. social fulfillment.
   c. feelings of usefulness.
   d. satisfaction and a sense of pride.
3. An elderly father moves in with his daughter and her family. He has many health problems. Which of the following statements is **TRUE**?
   a. The father may feel in control.
   b. The father and daughter may change roles.
   c. Tension may develop because of a lack of privacy.
   d. The father may feel a sense of dignity and self-respect.
4. Death of a spouse is a risk as people grow older. Which statement is **FALSE**?
   a. Men generally live longer than women.
   b. The surviving spouse may lose the will to live.
   c. The surviving spouse may develop serious physical problems.
   d. The surviving spouse may develop serious mental health problems.
5. Family and friends are important to residents for all of the following reasons except one. Which statement is **FALSE**?
   a. Their visits can help recovery.
   b. They offer comfort and support.
   c. They can help give care when the staff is busy.
   d. They help meet safety, security, love, and belonging needs.

SEXUALITY AND THE ELDERLY

Sexuality involves the whole personality, attitudes and feelings, as well as the body. The way a person behaves, thinks, dresses, and responds to others is related to that person's sexuality. Sexual relationships are as psychologically and physically important to the elderly as they are to younger persons. As the elderly person experiences other losses, feeling close to another human being may become important.

Illness, injury, and surgery may affect a person's sexuality. The problem may be temporary or permanent. The organs of reproduction, the circulatory system, or the nervous system may be affected. Changes also occur in the reproductive system as a result of aging. Elderly people may have sexual intercourse frequently, infrequently, or not at all. This does not mean they lack sexual needs or desires. Their needs may be expressed in other ways. Hand holding, touching, caressing, and embracing are ways of expressing closeness and intimacy. Respect for the person and understanding of these needs must always be conveyed. (TNA 659; LTCA 526–532)

Some persons may try to have their sexual needs met by health care workers. They may flirt, make sexual advances or comments, expose themselves, masturbate, or touch workers. Some sexually aggressive behaviors are a result of confusion or disorientation. The person may confuse the employee with his or her sexual partner. (TNA 661; LTCA 528–529)

Take note!

- Allow and encourage each person to practice grooming routines. Assist as needed. Let the person choose clothing and sleepwear.
- Do not expose the person unnecessarily. Screen and drape appropriately.
- Do not make judgments or gossip about the person's relationships.
- Provide privacy for those who wish to be alone with their partners. Arrange for roommates to be out of the room. Avoid interruptions.
- OBRA allows couples in long-term care facilities to share the same room if their conditions permit.
- Allow single elderly persons to develop new relationships.
- Sexual advances may be intentional. If the person becomes sexually aggressive, discuss the situation with the nurse. Ask the person not to touch you in places where you were touched. Explain to the person that his or her behavior makes you uncomfortable and politely ask him or her not to act that way.
- When the male becomes sexually aroused, the penis becomes enlarged, hard, and erect. In the female, the clitoris becomes enlarged and hard when sexually stimulated.
- If the person becomes sexually aroused or is masturbating, provide for safety (e.g., raise side rails, place the signal light within reach) and tell the person when you will return.

Questions for review (Answers to these questions are on page 87)

Circle the best answer.

1. Which of the following actions will **NOT** assist the resident with his or her sexuality?
   a. Allowing normal grooming routines
   b. Accepting the resident's relationship
   c. Having the resident wear a hospital gown
   d. Allowing the resident and his or her partner privacy
2. Illness and injury can cause impotence. Impotence is
   a. always permanent.
   b. the time when menstrual cycles stop.

c. the complete absence of sexual activity.
d. the inability of the male to achieve an erection.
3. Menopause is
   a. when menstruation stops.
   b. when a male is unable to have an erection.
   c. the physical activities involving the organs of reproduction.
   d. those physical, psychological, social, cultural, and spiritual factors that affect a person's feelings and attitudes about sex.
4. A resident is masturbating. You should
   a. tell the nurse.
   b. continue as if nothing has happened.
   c. provide for the resident's privacy and safety.
   d. tell the resident that his or her behavior makes you uncomfortable.
5. The following statements are about the resident's sexuality. Which one is **FALSE**?
   a. Knock before entering a resident's room.
   b. Allow residents to select their own clothing.
   c. Encourage residents to practice personal grooming routines.
   d. Residents should only be allowed to have sexual relationships with spouses.

THE DYING PERSON

Death can occur suddenly. Often it is expected. Many illnesses and diseases have no cure. Injuries can seriously affect the body's ability to function. Recovery is not expected in these cases.

The exact time of death cannot be predicted. It may come quickly or take weeks. Body processes slow, the person becomes weaker, and the level of consciousness decreases. Every effort is made to promote physical and psychological comfort. Doctors often write "do not resuscitate" orders for terminally ill persons so that no attempts will be made to resuscitate the person. The person is allowed to die in peace and dignity.

Five stages of dying have been identified by Dr. Elizabeth Kubler-Ross. These are: denial, anger, bargaining, depression, and acceptance. Dying persons do not always go through each stage. A person may never get beyond denial. Some move back and forth between stages. Listening and touch are very important ways to communicate with the dying person. Being there, helping, and sincerely caring about the person are what counts.

Spiritual needs of the dying person are important. Providing privacy when clergy visit, respecting religious objects, and letting the person participate in religious practices are ways to meet these needs.

As death approaches, vision blurs and eventually fails. Speech may be difficult. Hearing is usually intact until the moment of death. Body temperature rises and perspiration increases. Urinary and anal incontinence may occur. Pain is controlled with medication, positioning, and comfort measures.

Normal visiting hours do not apply. Family members are allowed to spend as much time as possible with the dying person. Remain courteous and supportive of the family during this difficult time. (TNA 711–721; LTCA 556–564)

Take note!

- Examine your own attitudes about death. Your feelings about death and dying affect the care you give.
- Always assume the dying or unconscious person can hear. Speak in a normal voice providing reassurance and explanations about care. Avoid topics that could upset the person.
- Provide oral hygiene as often as needed. Clean the mouth and nasal areas of mucus. Good skin care, bathing, and position changes promote comfort. Change linen and clothing as needed because of perspiration.
- Give perineal care as necessary. Watch for incontinence. Protect bed linens with waterproof bed protectors.
- Create a pleasant environment in the person's room. Keep it well lit. Remove unnecessary equipment. Eliminate odors as soon as possible.
- Absence of pulse, respirations, and blood pressure are signs of death. Pupils are fixed and dilated. A physician or nurse determines that death has occurred.
- Postmortem care is given after death to maintain the body's appearance. The care begins as soon as the doctor pronounces the person dead. Postmortem care involves positioning the body in normal alignment before rigor mortis sets in. The procedure differs with each facility. It always requires treating the body with dignity and respect.
- The family may want to see the body before it is taken to the morgue or funeral home. The body should appear to be in a comfortable and natural position for this viewing.

Questions for review (Answers to these questions are on page 88)

Circle the best answer.

1. An illness or injury for which there is no reasonable expectation of recovery is called a(n)
    a. acute illness.
    b. chronic illness.
    c. terminal illness.
    d. long-term illness.
2. As death approaches, the last sense to be lost is
    a. taste.
    b. sight.
    c. smell.
    d. hearing.
3. When a resident is dying, the family should
    a. not be allowed to provide resident care.
    b. be allowed to visit as often and as long as they want.
    c. be asked to leave as soon as visiting hours are over.
    d. be allowed to visit without interruptions for resident care.
4. A dying resident's speech is becoming very difficult to understand. You should
    a. avoid asking questions.
    b. tell the resident not to talk.
    c. ask the resident to write out messages.
    d. ask questions that can be answered with a "yes" or "no."
5. Which is **NOT** a sign death has occurred?
    a. No pulse
    b. The "death rattle"
    c. No respirations
    d. No blood pressure
6. As death approaches, movement, muscle tone, and sensation are lost. This usually begins in the
    a. arms.
    b. trunk.
    c. hands.
    d. feet and legs.
7. Mouth care for the dying resident is
    a. not necessary because the resident is not eating.
    b. only done if the resident appears uncomfortable.
    c. not done because it is painful and interrupts rest.
    d. done frequently because secretions tend to accumulate.
8. Rigor mortis usually occurs
    a. immediately after death.
    b. within 1 hour after death.
    c. 2 to 4 hours after death.
    d. 24 hours after death
9. Postmortem care is done
    a. after rigor mortis sets in.
    b. after the family has viewed the body.
    c. after the doctor pronounces the person dead.
    d. when the funeral director arrives for the body.
10. Persons in the stage of denial
    a. are angry.
    b. are sad and quiet.
    c. make "deals" with God.
    d. refuse to believe they are dying.

Chapter 4   *Safety*

WORDS TO REMEMBER

active physical restraint A restraint attached to the person's body and a stationary (nonmovable) object; movement and access to one's body are restricted

passive physical restraint A restraint near but not directly attached to the person's body; it does not totally restrict freedom of movement and allows access to certain body parts

restraint Any item, object, device, garment, material, or chemical that restricts a person's freedom of movement or access to one's body

THE SAFE ENVIRONMENT

A safe environment is one in which a person has a very low risk of illness or injury. The person feels safe both physically and psychologically. Surroundings are comfortable, well-lighted, and secure. (TNA 151–160; LTCA 112–131)

People cannot always protect themselves. Reasons include age, vision or hearing loss, limited movement, or medication. You need to promote a safe environment for the persons in your care. You need to identify each person before giving care. You need to take special precautions to prevent falls, burns, suffocation, and infection. Accidents need to be reported promptly according to facility policy. (TNA 151–160; LTCA 112–131)

Many elderly persons are at risk for accidents because of physical changes that occur as a result of aging. Movements are slower and less steady. Balance may be affected, causing the person to fall easily. The person may be unable to move quickly and suddenly to avoid dangerous situations. Other factors make elderly persons prone to accidents and injuries. These factors include decreased sensitivity to heat and cold, poor vision, hearing problems, and a decreased sense of smell. Confusion, poor judgment, memory problems, and disorientation are other factors. (TNA 152; LTCA 112)

Take note!

- Identify each person. Check identification bracelets (if worn) and call the person by name.
- Follow the facility's smoking regulations. Permit smoking only in designated areas.
- Check electrical equipment for frayed cords, improper operation, or poor connections. Do not use electric blankets, heating pads, or space heaters in the person's room.
- Check water temperature before the person enters the tub or shower.
- Cut food into small, bite-sized pieces for persons who cannot do so themselves. Immediately tell the nurse if a person is having difficulty swallowing.
- Do not leave a person alone in the bathtub.
- Move all persons from the area if you smell gas or smoke.
- Keep the person's bed in the lowest horizontal position except when giving bedside care. Use side rails as directed by the nurse.
- Falls are the most common accident in long-term care facilities. Suffocations, burns, and poisonings occur less often than falls.
- Keep floors free of spills and excess furniture and equipment.
- Have the person wear nonskid shoes or slippers when up. Check walkers, crutches, and canes for nonskid tips.
- Keep the person's signal light within reach at all times. Add nightlights during dark hours.
- Lock wheels of chairs, furniture, and equipment when transferring persons to and from them. Use transfer (gait) belts for ambulating and transferring persons.

- Accidents and errors are reported immediately to your supervisor. This includes accidents involving the person, visitors, or staff. You must report errors in care.
- Facilities require a written report about the accident or error. This is called an incident report. The report is completed as soon as possible after the accident or error.

Questions for review (Answers to these questions are on page 88)

Circle the best answer.

1. The most common accident in long-term care facilities is
   a. a fall.
   b. a burn.
   c. poisoning.
   d. suffocation.
2. Which of the following statements does **NOT** prevent burns?
   a. Banning smoking in bed
   b. Letting residents use heating pads during the daytime only
   c. Checking bath water temperature before the resident enters the tub
   d. Removing smoking materials from rooms of confused, disoriented, or drowsy residents
3. Which is a common cause of falls?
   a. Handrails
   b. Throw rugs
   c. Nonskid shoes and slippers
   d. Telephone and lamp at the bedside
4. The **BEST** way to identify a resident before giving care is to
   a. ask the nurse.
   b. call the resident by name.
   c. read the resident's identification bracelet.
   d. check the name on the door to the resident's room.
5. Which resident does **NOT** need to have the side rails raised?
   a. A confused resident
   b. A resident in a coma
   c. A resident sedated with medication
   d. A resident who is on self-care and who is aware of his surroundings
6. The following statements are about preventing falls. Which is **FALSE**?
   a. Residents should wear nonskid shoes when up.
   b. A nightlight should be kept on in the resident's room.
   c. The signal light should always be within the resident's reach.
   d. The bed should always be kept in the highest horizontal position.

7. You find a frayed electrical cord on a piece of equipment. You should
   a. change the cord.
   b. report it to the nurse.
   c. repair the item yourself.
   d. report it and continue to use the item.
8. You smell a strong gas odor in a resident's room. You should
   a. call the nurse.
   b. report the odor at the front desk.
   c. try to locate the source of the odor.
   d. remove the resident and yourself from the area.
9. You gave a treatment to the wrong resident. What should you do **FIRST**?
   a. Complete an incident report.
   b. Apologize to the resident involved.
   c. Give the treatment to the right resident.
   d. Immediately tell the nurse what happened.
10. Which resident is **LEAST** likely to be able to protect himself?
    a. Mr. McCabe who is 52 and in a coma.
    b. Mr. Jones who is 60 and wears glasses.
    c. Mr. Walker who is 80 and hard-of-hearing.
    d. Mr. Turner who is 71 and has a chest cold.

PROTECTIVE DEVICES (RESTRAINTS)

Restraints protect people from harming themselves or others. They prevent persons from falling out of beds or wheelchairs or off stretchers. Protective devices also prevent persons from crawling over side rails or the foot of the bed.

Restraints are for the person's protection, ***not*** for staff convenience. A doctor's order is required before a restraint can be used. The use of restraints unnecessarily is false imprisonment. Restraints must be applied correctly. The person needs special attention while protective devices are in place. Protective devices include: wrist and ankle restraints, mitt restraints, jacket (vest) restraints, and safety belts. (TNA 160–173; LTCA 116–127)

Take note!

- Position the person in good body alignment before applying the restraint. Pad bony areas and skin that may be injured by a restraint.
- Apply the restraint securely to protect the person, but allow some movement of the part. Make sure the person can breathe easily if the restraint involves the chest area.
- Tie restraints according to the facility policy. The policy should follow the manufacturer's instructions (Fig. 1). The knot must be easily released in an emergency. Quick-release knots

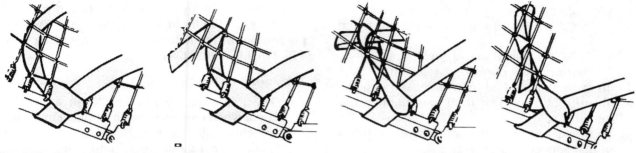

Fig. 1 The Posey quick-release tie. (From Sorrentino SA: *Mosby's Textbook for Nursing Assistants,* ed 4, St Louis, 1996, Mosby–Year Book.)

are often used. Some restraints have quick release buckles. Secure the restraint to the movable part of the bed frame or to the bed springs. Never secure the restraint to the side rails (Fig. 2). Make certain the person cannot reach the knot.

- Check the person's circulation every 15 to 30 minutes when using wrist or ankle restraints. Feel for a pulse at a pulse site below the restraint. Fingers and toes should be warm and pink in color.
- Remove the restraint and reposition the person every 2 hours. Give skin care and exercise the restrained part.
- Provide fluids and food as needed. Offer the bedpan and urinal every 2 hours. Always keep the signal light within the person's reach.
- The following information about restraints must be reported to the nurse:
  a. The type of restraint applied
  b. The time of application

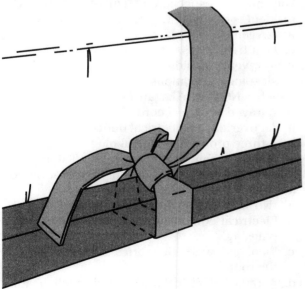

Fig. 2 The strap of the restraint is tied to the bed frame. (From Sorrentino SA: *Mosby's Textbook for Nursing Assistants,* ed 4, St Louis, 1996, Mosby–Year Book.)

  c. The time of removal
  d. The type of care given when the restraint was removed
  e. The color and condition of the person's skin
- Notify the nurse immediately if:
  a. You cannot feel a pulse
  b. Fingers or toes are cold, pale, or cyanotic (blue) in color
  c. The person complains of pain, numbness, or tingling in the restrained part
  d. The skin is red or damaged

Skills list

Applying a Jacket or Vest Restraint, page 112

Questions for review (Answers to these questions are on page 89)

Circle the best answer.

1. Which statement about restraints is **FALSE**?
   a. Restraints require a doctor's order.
   b. A restraint should prevent all movement of the body part.
   c. Bony areas need to be padded when a restraint is applied.
   d. A resident may become more confused and agitated after restraints are applied.
2. Which does **NOT** need to be reported to the nurse?
   a. The time the restraints were applied
   b. The reason the restraints were applied
   c. The type of restraint applied
   d. The care given when the restraints were removed
3. The restraint is removed and the resident repositioned every
   a. 15 minutes.
   b. hour.
   c. 2 hours.
   d. 4 hours.
4. Notify the nurse immediately if
   a. the restraint is secured to the bed frame.
   b. the resident is having difficulty breathing.

c. the resident keeps pulling at the restraint.

d. the resident's fingers and toes are warm and pink.

5. Which is **NOT** a reason to use a restraint?

   a. To control an uncooperative resident

   b. To prevent a resident from falling out of bed

   c. To prevent a resident from harming himself/herself

   d. To prevent a resident from pulling out tubes or disconnecting equipment

6. You are to apply a jacket restraint. Which is **FALSE**?

   a. Apply the restraint over the resident's clothing.

   b. Apply the vest so the straps cross in the back.

   c. Tie the straps to the bed frame with a square knot.

   d. Make sure the resident is comfortable and in good body alignment.

7. A resident complains of numbness and tingling in the restrained part. You should

   a. remove the restraint.

   b. reposition the resident.

   c. tell the nurse immediately.

   d. reassure the resident and explain why the restraint is needed.

8. In order to promote a resident's quality of life,

   a. the restraints should be used for as long as possible.

   b. the care plan should show how the use of restraints should slowly be increased.

   c. you should not exercise the resident's joints because they need to rest as much as possible.

   d. you should remove the restraint, give skin care, and reposition the resident every 2 hours.

FIRE SAFETY

Fire safety is the responsibility of the entire health care team. You must know what to do if there is a fire. It is imperative that you know the location of fire alarms, fire extinguishers, and emergency exits.

Remember that if oxygen is being used, special fire precautions must be followed. Smoking is not allowed in any area where oxygen is in use or stored. This rule applies to the person, visitors, and staff. Smoking is allowed only in specified areas. If allowed to smoke, the person must be supervised.

You must be able to act if there is a fire or fire drill. By remembering the word RACE, you will be able to respond to a fire or fire drill appropriately.

Rescue whoever is in immediate danger.

Alert the facility by sounding the nearest fire alarm.

Confine the fire by closing all doors and windows.

Extinguish the fire if it is a small fire or **E**vacuate persons in the immediate area to a safe place. (TNA 175–176; LTCA 129–130)

Take note!

- The following are removed from a person's room when oxygen is used: smoking materials, matches, lighters, electrical equipment, wool blankets, synthetic fibers, and flammable materials (such as oil, grease, alcohol, and nail polish remover).

- Faulty electrical equipment and wiring, overloaded electrical circuits, and smoking are major causes of fire.

- If a fire is discovered, rescue whoever is in immediate danger. Sound the nearest alarm. Then alert the facility of the exact location according to the facility procedure. Move persons in the immediate area of the fire to a safe place.

- Close all doors and windows. Clear hallways and emergency exits of equipment. Turn off oxygen and electrical equipment being used in the area of the fire.

- Use a fire extinguisher on a small fire that has not spread. Remove the safety pin, push down on the top handle, and aim the hose at the base of the fire.

- Do not use elevators if there is a fire.

Questions for review (Answers to these questions are on page 89)

Circle the best answer.

1. You must be especially careful about fire if the resident is receiving

   a. oxygen.

   b. heat treatments.

   c. intravenous fluids.

   d. sleeping medications.

2. Which is **NOT** a fire hazard?

   a. A frayed electrical cord

   b. An overloaded electrical outlet

   c. A three-pronged electrical plug

   d. Electrical equipment that gives off shocks

3. A resident is receiving oxygen. Which of the following nursing actions is **INCORRECT**?

   a. "No smoking" is strictly enforced.

   b. Electrical equipment is turned off before unplugging.

   c. Wool and synthetic fabrics are removed from the room.

   d. A radio, electrical razor, and small heating pad may be used by the resident with caution.

4. The fire alarm rings in the facility. What should you do first?

   a. Locate the fire.

   b. Pull the closest alarm.

c. Take a fire extinguisher to the scene.

d. Move all residents out of the building.

5. The fire alarm has sounded. Which action is **WRONG**?

   a. Clear all exits of equipment.

   b. Close all windows and doors.

   c. Move all residents to the lobby.

   d. Do not let visitors use the elevator.

6. You are using a fire extinguisher. The hose is aimed at the

   a. top of the flame.

   b. middle of the flame.

   c. base of the fire.

   d. area around the fire.

Chapter 5   *Infection control*

WORDS TO REMEMBER

asepsis Being free of disease-producing microorganisms

bacteria Microscopic plant life that multiply rapidly; they consist of one cell and are often called *germs*

biohazardous waste Items contaminated with blood, body fluids, or body substances and that may be harmful to others; *bio* means life and *hazardous* means dangerous or harmful

carrier A human being or animal that is a reservoir for microorganisms but does not have signs and symptoms of infection

clean technique Medical asepsis

communicable disease A disease caused by pathogens that are easily spread; a contagious disease

contact precautions Prevent the spread of infection by close or direct contact

contagious disease Communicable disease

contamination The process by which an object or area becomes unclean

disinfection The process by which pathogens are destroyed

enteric precautions Prevent the spread of pathogens through feces (bowel movement)

host The environment in which microorganisms live and grow; reservoir

immunity Protection against a specific disease

infection A disease state that results from the invasion and growth of microorganisms in the body

medical asepsis The practices used to remove or destroy pathogens and to prevent their spread from one person or place to another person or place; clean technique

microorganism A small *(micro)* living plant or animal *(organism)* that cannot be seen without the the aid of a microscope; a microbe; they need a reservoir to live and grow

nosocomial infection An infection acquired after admission to a health care facility

nonpathogen A microorganism that does not usually cause an infection

pathogen A microorgansim that is harmful and capable of causing an infection

personal protective equipment Specialized clothing or equipment (gloves, gown, mask, goggles, face shield) worn for protection against a hazard

protozoa Microscopic one-celled animals

reservoir The environment in which microorganisms live and grow; the host; it can be a person, a plant, an animal, the soil, food, water, or other material

respiratory precautions Prevent the spread of pathogens through airborne droplets

spore A bacterium protected by a hard shell that forms around the microorganism

surgical asepsis The practices that keep equipment and supplies free of all microorganisms; sterile technique

sterile The absence of all microorganisms

sterile technique Surgical asepsis

sterilization The process by which all microorganisms are destroyed

universal precautions Involve setting up barriers to prevent contact with blood, body fluids, or body substances

MEDICAL ASEPSIS

The term "medical asepsis" refers to the techniques and practices used to prevent the spread of disease-causing microorganisms (pathogens). Medical asepsis (clean technique) is different from sterilization. Some common daily practices are aseptic techniques. These include bathing, handwashing after urinating or having a bowel movement, handwashing when preparing food, and providing individual toothbrushes and towels.

Microorganisms are everywhere. They can be seen only with a microscope. Many microorganisms are harmless. Others can cause disease and are called pathogens. These must be controlled or eliminated.

Handwashing with soap and water is one of the easiest and most important ways to prevent the spread of infection. The technique must be done correctly and frequently to be effective. Equipment used in the person's care must be cleaned properly. Other aseptic measures include cleaning from the cleanest to the dirtiest areas, not sitting on a person's bed, and not sharing equipment between persons. (TNA 186–191; LTCA 136–143)

Take note!

- Handwashing is the single most effective means of preventing the spread of infection.
- When handwashing, use warm running water and soap. Stand away from the sink so your clothes do not touch the sink. Hold hands and forearms lower than the elbows throughout the procedure. Use a clean, dry paper towel to turn off the faucets. Be sure to clean under the fingernails.
- Guidelines for handwashing:
  - 2 minutes before caring for any person at the beginning of your shift
  - 10 to 15 seconds before caring for another person
  - 1 minute or longer if your hands are contaminated with blood, body fluids, or a body substance
  - 1 to 2 minutes if you have given care to a person with an infection
- Rinse equipment in cold water first to remove organic material. Then wash in soap and hot water. Use a brush if necessary. Rinse and dry the equipment. Disinfect or sterilize equipment according to the facility's guidelines.
- Hold linens and equipment away from your uniform. Clean away from your body and uniform.
- Avoid shaking linens and other equipment.

Skills list

Handwashing, page 111

Questions for review (Answers to these questions are on page 90)

Circle the best answer.

1. A microorganism needs the following to grow **EXCEPT**
   a. food.
   b. light.
   c. water.
   d. warmth.
2. A microorganism that can cause an infection is called a
   a. pathogen.
   b. protozoa.
   c. bacteria.
   d. nonpathogen.
3. The practices that prevent the spread of pathogens from one person or place to another are called
   a. sterilization.
   b. handwashing.
   c. contamination.
   d. medical asepsis.
4. An object or area becomes unclean. This is called
   a. sterilization.
   b. disinfection.
   c. contamination.
   d. medical asepsis.
5. All microorganisms are destroyed. This process is
   a. sterilization.
   b. disinfection.
   c. contamination.
   d. medical asepsis.
6. You are going to wash your hands. You should stand
   a. right up against the sink.
   b. 6 inches away from the sink.
   c. 2 feet away from the sink.
   d. far enough away so that your uniform does not touch the sink.
7. You should wash your hands for approximately
   a. 1 to 2 minutes.
   b. 4 minutes.
   c. 6 minutes.
   d. 8 minutes.

8. After drying your hands, you should
    a. turn off the faucet.
    b. throw the paper towel away.
    c. clean the sink with paper towels.
    d. turn off the faucet with a clean, dry paper towel.
9. You are going to clean a bedpan. Which should you do **FIRST**?
    a. Rinse the bedpan with cold water.
    b. Use a brush to clean the bedpan.
    c. Wash the bedpan with hot water and soap.
    d. Ask the nurse if you should clean the bedpan.
10. Handwashing is an example of
    a. sterilization.
    b. disinfection.
    c. contamination.
    d. medical asepsis.

COMMUNICABLE DISEASE CONTROL

Communicable (contagious) diseases can be spread from one person to another. Infection precautions must be taken when certain pathogens are present or suspected.

Infection precautions are used for persons with highly contagious respiratory, wound, skin, gastrointestinal, or blood infections. These techniques are sometimes used to protect persons who are very susceptible to infection. This may be a result of age, weakness, illness, or certain medications. (TNA 192; LCTA 142)

Universal precautions were issued by the Centers for Disease Control (CDC) in 1987 to prevent the spread of bloodborne pathogens. **Universal precautions are used for ALL persons.** Universal precautions involve setting up barriers to prevent contact with blood, body fluids, or body substances. Routine use of barrier precautions (gloves) prevents the caregiver from exposure to blood or body fluids. (TNA 192; LTCA 143)

Isolation precautions prevent the spread of pathogens from one area to another. Barriers are set up to prevent the spread of pathogens. By using special procedures (based on how the pathogen is spread), the pathogens are kept within a specific area, usually the person's room. When isolation precautions are ordered, the person is separated from others. A private room is preferred. If necessary, a semiprivate room is used. The room must have a sink with running water. Equipment for measuring temperature, pulse, respiration, and blood pressure is kept in the room. In addition to the waste basket, there are containers for laundry and trash.

There is a cabinet, bedside stand, or cart outside the room. This is used to store supplies needed for isolation precautions: gowns, gloves, masks, pro-

tective eyewear, plastic bags, laundry bags, and trash bags. A sign is placed on the outside of the room door. It states the precautions being practiced.

Gloves Disposable gloves act as a barrier between the person and the nursing assistant. Gloves protect the nursing assistant from pathogens in the person's blood, body fluids, and body substances. The person is also protected from microorganisms that may be on the nursing assistant's hands.

Gloves are worn whenever contact with blood or body fluids, body substances, or mucous membranes that contain blood or are infected may occur. This includes saliva, vomitus, urine, feces, vaginal discharge, mucus, semen, wound drainage, pus, and respiratory secretions.

When wearing gloves:
* A new pair is needed for every person.
* Torn, cut, or punctured gloves are removed immediately and discarded. Wash your hands and put on a new pair.
* Gloves are worn once and discarded.
* New gloves are needed whenever gloves become contaminated with infective material. More than one pair of gloves may be needed for a procedure.
* Gloves are pulled up to cover the wrists. If a gown is worn, the gloves must cover the cuffs.
* When gloves are removed, the inside part will be on the outside. The inside of the gloves is considered *clean.* (TNA 196–198; LTCA 144–145)

Gowns Gowns keep clothing free from the person's pathogenic microorganisms. Gowns also protect the person from microbes that may be on the clothing of staff and visitors who enter the room. They also prevent soiling of clothing when giving care. Gowns are never worn outside the person's room.

When gowns are worn:
* The gown must be long enough and large enough to cover clothing completely
* The sleeves are long with tight cuffs
* The gown opens at the back, where it is tied at the neck and waist
* The inside and neck of the gown are clean
* The outside and waist strings are contaminated
* It is considered contaminated when it becomes wet; remove the wet gown and put on a dry one (TNA 199; LTCA 146)

Face mask Face masks prevent the spread of microbes from the respiratory tract. Masks may be worn by the person, visitors, or health care workers. If a mask becomes wet or moist from breathing, it is contaminated. A new mask is applied when contamination occurs.

When masks are worn:

- The mask should be snug over the nose and mouth.
- The hands are washed before putting on a mask.
- Remove your gloves and wash your hands before untying the strings.
- Only the strings are touched during removal; the front of the mask is considered contaminated. (TNA 148–149; LTCA 200–201)

Protective eyewear Goggles or face shields are worn when splashing or splattering is likely. They are worn with face masks. Together the mask and protective eyewear protect your eyes, nose, and mouth from splashing or splattering blood or oral fluids. Disposable eyewear is discarded after use. Reusable eyewear is cleaned before being used for another person. It is washed with soap and water and then a facility-approved disinfectant is used. (TNA 201; LTCA 148)

Take note!

- Floors are contaminated. Any object on the floor or that falls on the floor is contaminated.
- Prevent drafts. Pathogens are carried in the air by drafts.
- Do not touch your hair, nose, mouth, eyes, or other body parts when caring for a person. If your hands become contaminated, do not touch any clean area or object. Wash your hands immediately.
- Place clean items on paper towels. Turn faucets on and off with paper towels.
- Tell the nurse if you have any cuts, open skin areas, sore throat, vomiting, or diarrhea.
- Gowns must be long enough to cover your clothing completely. They should have long sleeves with tight cuffs. A wet gown is considered contaminated. Remove it and put on a dry one.
- Isolation precautions may require wearing gloves, a gown, a mask, or protective eyewear.
- Double bagging may be needed when removing linens, trash, or equipment from the area.
- Items removed from the isolation room are bagged and labeled.
- Special measures are needed to collect specimens and to transport persons on isolation precautions.
- Blood or other specimens are clearly labeled with "Blood/Body Fluid Precautions." Specimens are placed in appropriate containers or bags to prevent leaks during transport.
- Blood or body fluids spills are cleaned up promptly. Use a facility-approved disinfectant. Nondisposable items contaminated with blood or body fluids are washed with the solution before being sterilized.

- Isolation precautions may require wearing gloves, a gown, a mask, or protective eyewear.
- Double bagging may be needed when removing linens, trash, or equipment from the area.
- Items removed from the isolation room are bagged and labeled.
- Special measures are needed to collect specimens and to transport persons on isolation precautions.

Skills list

Universal Precautions, page 107

Questions for review (Answers to these questions are on page 90)

Circle the best answer.

1. Isolation precautions are used for residents with
   a. allergies.
   b. contagious diseases.
   c. any type of infection.
   d. gastrointestinal diseases.
2. Drainage/secretion precautions are ordered for a resident with a draining pressure ulcer. You need to wear
   a. a mask at all times.
   b. a gown at all times.
   c. gloves at all times.
   d. a gown and gloves if you have direct contact with the wound or drainage.
3. Pathogens spread through fecal material are controlled with
   a. enteric precautions.
   b. contact precautions.
   c. universal precautions.
   d. respiratory precautions.
4. Respiratory isolation is ordered. This prevents the spread of pathogens through
   a. feces.
   b. airborne droplets.
   c. wounds or drainage.
   d. direct or indirect contact with blood or body fluids.
5. Infection precautions are ordered. You should do all of the following **EXCEPT**
   a. place clean items or objects on paper towels.
   b. wash your hands if they become contaminated.
   c. bag linens, equipment, and garbage before leaving the room.
   d. use paper towels to handle contaminated equipment and objects.
6. What should you do **FIRST** when putting on a gown?
   a. Tie the waist strings.
   b. Tie the strings at the neck.

c. Overlap the back of the gown.

d. Make sure it completely covers all of your uniform.

7. What should you do **FIRST** when removing a gown?

a. Wash your hands.

b. Untie the neck strings.

c. Untie the waist strings.

d. Pull the gown down from the shoulders.

8. Universal precautions are used for

a. all residents.

b. residents with AIDS only.

c. residents who have infections.

d. residents who have blood disorders.

9. Infection precautions

a. prevent infection.

b. destroy pathogens.

c. destroy pathogens and nonpathogens.

d. keep pathogens within a specific area.

10. Items that are contaminated with the resident's blood, body fluids, or body substances are referred to as

a. normal trash.

b. normal waste.

c. biohazardous waste.

d. biodegradable waste.

Chapter 6 — *The person's comfort*

WORDS TO REMEMBER

base of support The area on which an object rests

body alignment The way in which body parts are aligned with one another; posture

body mechanics Using the body in an efficient and careful way

closed bed A bed that is not being used by the person; also, one that is ready for a new person; the top linens are not folded back

dangling Sitting on the side of the bed; sitting on the side of the bed and moving the legs back and forth and around in circles

dorsal recumbent position The back-lying or supine position

drawsheet A small sheet placed over the middle of the bottom sheet; it helps keep the mattress and bottom linens clean and dry and can be used to turn and move the person in bed; the cotton drawsheet

Fowler's position A semi-sitting position; the head of the bed is elevated 45 to 60 degrees

friction The rubbing of one surface against another

gait belt A transfer belt

lateral position The side-lying position

logrolling Turning the person as a unit in alignment with one motion

mitered corner A way of tucking linens under the mattress to help keep them straight and smooth

occupied bed A bed that is made with the person in it

open bed A bed that is being used by the person; the top linens are folded back so that the person can get into bed; a closed bed becomes an open bed when the top linens are folded back

plastic drawsheet A drawsheet made of plastic; it is placed between the bottom sheet and the cotton drawsheet to keep the mattress and bottom linens clean and dry

posture The way in which body parts are aligned with one another; body alignment

reverse Trendelenburg's position The head of the bed is raised, and the foot of the bed is lowered

semi-Fowler's position The head of the bed is raised 45 degrees, and the knee portion is raised 15 degrees; or the head of the bed is raised 30 degrees

shearing When skin sticks to a surface and the muscles slide in the direction the body is moving

side-lying The lateral position

Sims' position A side-lying position in which the upper leg is sharply flexed so that it is not on the lower leg and the lower arm is behind the person

supine position The back-lying or dorsal recumbent position

surgical bed A bed that is made so the person can be moved from a stretcher to the bed; it may be called a postoperative bed, recovery bed, or anesthetic bed

transfer belt A belt used to hold onto a person during a transfer or when walking with the person; a gait belt

Trendelenburg's position The head of the bed is lowered, and the foot of the bed is raised

unoccupied bed May be either a closed or an open bed

THE PATIENT/RESIDENT UNIT

The person's unit is the furniture and equipment provided for the individual by the health care facility.

It is designed and equipped to meet the person's basic needs. Age, illness, and activity affect comfort. Factors like temperature, lighting, ventilation, noise, and odors are controlled for the person's comfort. Curtains and screens provide privacy. A telephone, television, and radio help the person keep in touch with family, friends, and the world. (TNA 253–262; LTCA 194–199)

A temperature range of 68° to 74° F is usually comfortable for most healthy people. The elderly and chronically ill persons generally need higher room temperatures for comfort. OBRA requires that nursing facilities maintain a temperature range of 71° to 81° F. (TNA 253–254; LTCA 194)

Many odors occur in health care facilities. Good nursing care, good ventilation, and good housekeeping practices help eliminate unpleasant odors. Nursing personnel can reduce odors by:

- Checking incontinent persons often
- Emptying and washing bedpans and emesis basins promptly
- Changing soiled linens or clothing promptly
- Changing and washing incontinent persons promptly
- Providing individuals with good personal hygiene to prevent body and breath odors
- Using a room deodorizer when necessary and if allowed by the facility; do not use spray deodorizers around persons with breathing problems

Common health care sounds are disturbing. When in a strange place, people want to know the cause and meaning of new sounds. This is part of the basic need to feel safe and secure. Staff can reduce noise by controlling the loudness of their voices and handling equipment carefully. Keeping

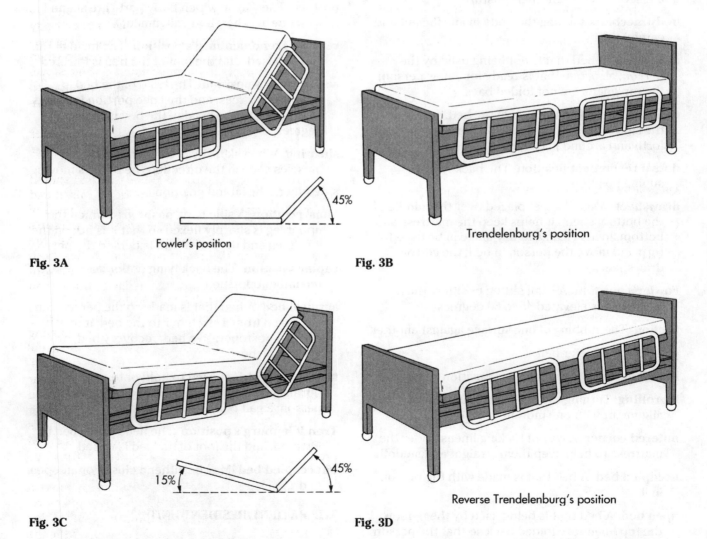

Fowler's position

Fig. 3A

45%

Trendelenburg's position

Fig. 3B

15%   45%

Fig. 3C

Reverse Trendelenburg's position

Fig. 3D

Fig. 3 A, Fowler's position, **B,** Trendelenburg's position, **C,** semi-Fowler's position, **D,** reverse Trendelenburg's position. (From Sorrentino SA: *Mosby's Textbook for Nursing Assistants,* ed 4, St Louis, 1996, Mosby–Year Book.)

equipment working properly and promptly answering telephones and intercoms also decrease noise. (TNA 254; LTCA 194–195)

Good lighting is needed for the safety and comfort of the person and staff. Glares, shadows, and dull lighting can cause falls, headaches, and eyestrain. Dim lighting allows the person to relax and rest better. A bright room is cheerful and stimulating. Bright lighting is helpful when care is given. Light controls should be within the person's reach. (TNA 254; LTCA 195–196)

Take note!

- Make sure the person can reach the overbed table and bedside stand. Arrange personal belongings as desired by the person.
- Keep the signal light within reach at all times.
- Provide enough toilet tissue, tissues, paper towels, and other necessities. Adjust room lighting, temperature, and ventilation for the person's comfort.
- Handle equipment carefully to prevent unnecessary noise. Explain the causes of strange noises to the person.
- Use room deodorizers and empty wastebaskets as needed.
- Know how to operate manual and electric beds. Know the four basic bed positions—Fowler's, semi-Fowler's, Trendelenburg's, and reverse Trendelenburg's (Fig. 3).

Questions for review (Answers to these questions are on page 91)

Circle the best answer.

1. A resident in a wheelchair complains of a draft. Your best action would be to
   a. return the resident to bed.
   b. bring the resident a lap robe.
   c. close off the air vent near the resident.
   d. move the resident to a draft-free location.
2. OBRA requires that nursing facilities maintain a temperature of
   a. 65° to 70° F.
   b. 68° to 72° F.
   c. 70° to 78° F.
   d. 71° to 81° F.
3. A resident needs to rest and relax. Room lighting should be
   a. dim.
   b. soft.
   c. natural sunlight.
   d. very bright and cheerful.
4. Noise can be controlled by all of the following **EXCEPT**
   a. handling equipment carefully.
   b. answering call lights promptly.

c. controlling the loudness of your voice.
d. playing music over the intercom system.
5. The head of the bed is elevated on blocks and the foot is lowered. This position is called
   a. Fowler's.
   b. semi-Fowler's.
   c. Trendelenburg's.
   d. reverse Trendelenburg's.

BODY MECHANICS

Body mechanics is using the body in an efficient and careful way. It involves using good posture, balance, and the body's strongest and largest muscles to perform work. You need to be concerned about this for yourself and the person. A good base of support is essential to maintain balance. Learn to use the larger muscles of your shoulders, upper arms, hips, and thighs when lifting. (TNA 213; LTCA 158–159)

Some persons cannot move or turn in bed by themselves. Remember the principles of good body mechanics when moving, lifting, or transferring persons. Always try to reduce the friction created when the person's skin rubs against linen during movement. A turning sheet should be used. Remember to ask other workers to help you when the person cannot help in moving. (TNA 218–226; LTCA 160–173)

There are many ways to move, turn, and transfer persons. Each procedure involves good body mechanics and proper alignment of the person.

When moving a person up in bed, the bed should be as flat as possible. The far side rail is raised and the one nearest you is lowered. Facing the head of the bed, one arm is placed under the person's shoulders and the other under the thighs. Ask the person to grasp the headboard and to flex both knees. Ask the person to pull on the headboard with the hands and push against the bed with the feet on the count of "3." (TNA 223–224; LTCA 164–165)

At least two people are needed to move heavy persons or those weak from disease. When moving a person up in bed with the assistance of a co-worker, you should flatten the bed as much as possible. You stand on one side of the bed while your co-worker stands on the other side. Both of you should place one arm under the person's shoulder and one arm under the buttocks. Grasp each other's forearms. Move the person to the head of the bed on the count of "3." (TNA 224–225; LTCA 166)

Lifting sheets (turning sheets) can be used to help you and a co-worker easily and safely move a person up in bed. Friction and shearing are reduced, and the person is lifted more evenly. A flat sheet folded in half or a drawsheet is used for the lift sheet. The lift sheet is placed under the person, extending from the shoulders to above the knees.

The rolled-up lifting sheet is grasped firmly near the shoulders and buttocks. (TNA 226–227; LTCA 167)

Persons are moved to the side of the bed for repositioning and for certain procedures such as a bed bath. The bed should be as flat as possible. The far side rail is raised and the one near you is lowered. Cross the person's arms over the person's chest. Move the person in segments, beginning with the person's neck and shoulders. Then the person's waist and thighs are moved. The legs and feet are moved last. (TNA 228–229; LTCA 168–169)

People are helped to sit on the side of the bed (dangle) for many reasons. Many elderly persons become dizzy or faint if they get out of bed too fast. They may need to sit on the side of the bed for 1 to 5 minutes before walking or transferring. Two workers may be needed to help the person dangle. The person should lie down if a feeling of faintness occurs. Certain observations are made while the person is sitting on the side of the bed:

- Take pulse and respirations
- Observe for difficulty in breathing
- Observe for pallor of cyanosis
- Note complaints of dizziness or lightheadedness (TNA 233–235; LTCA 174–175)

A transfer belt (gait belt) is used when transferring persons who need assistance. The belt goes around the person's waist over clothing. It is not applied over bare skin. The belt is tightened so that it is snug. It should not cause discomfort or impair breathing. Make sure that a woman's breasts are not caught under the belt. The buckle is placed either off center in the front or in the back for the person's comfort. The belt is grasped to support the person during the transfer.

Safety is very important when transferring a person to a chair or wheelchair. Falls must be prevented. The person is helped out of bed on his or her strong side. When transferring, the strong side moves first and pulls the weaker side along. The nurse may ask you to take the person's pulse before and after the transfer. The pulse rate gives some information about how the activity was tolerated. Report the amount of help needed and how the person helped in the transfer. Also observe and report if the person:

- Tires easily
- Complains of weakness or being lightheaded
- Has pain or discomfort
- Has difficulty breathing (dyspnea) (TNA 237–238; LTCA 177–179)

Mechanical lifts can be used to transfer helpless persons. Be certain you know how to operate the lift properly and that it is in good working condition. At least two people are needed to transfer a person with a mechanical lift. The manufacturer's instructions are followed for a safe transfer. (TNA 242–244; LTCA 182–183)

Persons are transferred to stretchers for transport within the facility or to another facility. A drawsheet can be used to transfer a person from the bed to a stretcher. At least three workers are needed for a safe transfer. Safety straps are used when the person is on the stretcher. The stretcher's side rails are kept up during the transport. Move the person feet first so the co-worker at the head of the stretcher can watch the person's breathing and color during the transport. A person on a stretcher is never left unattended. (TNA 245; LTCA 184–185)

Correct positioning in bed or in a chair promotes comfort and well-being. Complications can be prevented through frequent position changes. The basic positions for the person in bed are: Fowler's, supine, prone, lateral, and Sims'.

Fowler's position Good alignment for Fowler's position involves keeping the spine straight, supporting the head with a small pillow, and supporting the arms with pillows. A small pillow may be placed under the lower back. Small pillows may also be placed under the thighs and ankles.

Supine position Good alignment for the supine position involves having the bed flat, supporting the head and shoulders on a pillow, and placing the arms and hands at the person's sides. The arms may be supported with regular-size pillows. The hands may be supported on small pillows with the palms down. A small pillow may be placed under the ankles. A folded or rolled towel may be placed under the lower part of the back. A small pillow may be placed under the person's thighs, if requested.

Prone position Position the person in the prone position by placing a small pillow under the head, one under the abdomen, and one under the lower legs. The arms are flexed at the elbows with the hands near the head. Persons may be positioned with their feet hanging over the end of the mattress. If that is done, a pillow is not needed under the lower legs. Most elderly persons do not tolerate the prone position well because of limited range of motion in their necks.

Lateral position Good alignment for the lateral position includes placing a pillow under the head and neck and supporting the upper leg and thigh with pillows. A small pillow is placed under the upper hand and arm, and a pillow is positioned against the person's back.

Sims' position Good alignment in the Sims' position involves placing a pillow under the person's head and neck, supporting the upper leg with a pillow, and placing a pillow under the upper arm and hand. (TNA 246–249; LTCA 186–188)

Persons who sit in chairs must be able to hold their upper bodies and heads erect. The person's back and buttocks are against the back of the chair. Feet are flat on the floor or on the wheelchair footrests. Backs of the knees and calves are slightly away from the edge of the seat. With the nurse's permission, a small pillow may be placed between the person's lower back and the chair. (Note: A pillow is not placed behind the back if restraints are used.) Paralyzed arms are positioned on pillows. Wrists are positioned at a slight upward angle. Postural supports and positioners may be needed to keep the person in good body alignment. Sometimes restraints are used for postural support. The rules and safety measures for restraints apply when they are used as postural supports. (TNA 249–250; LTCA 189)

Take note!

- Maintain a wide base of support. Stand with your feet about 12 inches apart. Hold objects close to your body when lifting, moving, or carrying them. Keep your palms up and stand close to your work area. It should be level with your waist, if possible.
- Push, slide, or pull to avoid lifting. Do not twist your back or neck. Avoid sudden, jerky movements. Get help in lifting.
- Decide how you will move a person and if you will need help. Encourage the person to help when possible. Be gentle. Avoid touching tender or painful areas.
- Get enough co-workers to help you before beginning the procedure.
- Use cautions when moving persons with severe arthritis or osteoporosis. Always ask for help when moving them to avoid causing pain or injury.
- Protect any tubes or drainage containers when moving a person.
- Keep the person covered and screened to protect the right to privacy.
- When transferring a person, arrange the room so there is enough space. Place the chair or wheelchair correctly for a safe and easy transfer.
- Make sure the person is wearing nonskid shoes or slippers. Explain what you are going to do. Let the person help when possible.
- Use a gait (transfer) belt when working with a helpless or semi-helpless person. Apply the belt around the person's waist.
- Make sure all wheels of beds, stretchers, and wheelchairs are locked in place before use.

Skills list

Questions for review (Answers to these questions are on page 91)

Circle the best answer.

1. Weak and small muscle groups are located in the
   a. hips.
   b. thighs.
   c. back.
   d. shoulders and upper arms.
2. An object is very heavy. You should **NOT**
   a. lift it.
   b. pull it.
   c. push it.
   d. slide it.
3. You are going to move a resident up in bed. The bed should be
   a. as flat as possible.
   b. raised at the foot.
   c. raised at the head.
   d. in the low horizontal position.
4. You are going to move a resident up in bed with assistance. Your co-worker should stand
   a. at the foot of the bed.
   b. at the head of the bed.
   c. on the same side of the bed as you.
   d. on the side of the bed opposite you.
5. You are going to use a turning sheet to turn a resident. Grasp the sheet at the
   a. waist and knees.
   b. shoulders and waist.
   c. shoulders and knees.
   d. shoulders and buttocks.
6. You are going to move a resident to the side of the bed. You should **NOT**
   a. raise the side rail on your side.
   b. cross the resident's arms over his or her chest.
   c. move the resident in segments beginning with the neck and shoulders.
   d. stand on the side of the bed to which you will be moving the resident.
7. Logrolling involves
   a. using a mechanical lift.
   b. always using a turning sheet.
   c. moving the resident in segments.
   d. turning the resident over in one motion.
8. Which is the proper placement of your arms when moving a resident up in bed?
   a. Slide your arms under the resident's arms.
   b. Place one arm under the resident's waist and the other under the thighs.

    c. Place one arm under the resident's shoulders and the other under the thighs.

    d. Place one arm under the resident's waist and the other under the shoulders.

9. A resident is being transported on a stretcher. Which is **FALSE**?
    a. Safety straps are applied.
    b. The resident is moved feet first.
    c. The side rails are kept up when transporting the resident.
    d. The resident can be left alone if the safety straps are in place.

10. How many people are needed to safely transfer a resident on a stretcher to the bed?
    a. 1
    b. 2
    c. 3
    d. 4

11. You are going to assist a resident to stand using a transfer belt. You should do all of the following **EXCEPT**
    a. tighten the belt so it is snug.
    b. apply the belt over bare skin.
    c. place the buckle off center in the front.
    d. make sure the belt does not impair breathing.

12. A resident is to be transferred from a bed to a chair. The resident should be helped out of bed on the
    a. left side of the bed.
    b. person's weak side.
    c. person's strong side.
    d. right side of the bed.

13. A resident is dangling at the bedside. You observe that the resident has cyanosis, is pale, and is having difficulty breathing. What should you do?
    a. Return the resident to a lying position.
    b. Immediately report your observations to the nurse.
    c. Encourage the resident to take a few deep breaths.
    d. Ask the resident to push both fists into the mattress for support.

14. Another name for the supine position is
    a. Sims' position.
    b. prone position.
    c. Fowler's position.
    d. dorsal recumbent position.

15. In the lateral position, do **NOT** place a pillow
    a. against the back.
    b. under the lower legs.
    c. under the upper leg and thigh.
    d. under the resident's head and shoulders.

16. Which is **NOT** good positioning in a chair?
    a. Feet are flat on the floor.
    b. Calves are against the seat.
    c. Back and buttocks are against the chair.
    d. Backs of the knees are slightly away from the seat.

BEDMAKING

Clean and neat beds help persons feel more comfortable. Keeping the bed clean, dry, and wrinkle-free helps prevent skin breakdown. In nursing facilities, a complete linen change is done on the person's bath day or as needed. Linens are straightened if they become loose and wrinkled during the day. Check linens for crumbs after meals and properly remove them. Also straighten linens at bedtime. Linens are changed whenever they become wet, soiled, or damp. Closed, occupied, and surgical beds are made.

Linens must be handled according to the principles of medical asepsis. Your uniform is considered dirty. Always hold linens away from your body and uniform. Never shake linens in the air since shaking them causes the spread of microbes. Clean linens are placed on a clean surface. Never put dirty linen on the floor.

To remove dirty linens from the bed, roll the linens away from you so that the side that touched the person is inside the roll. Not all linens are changed every time the bed is made. They are reused for an open bed if they are not soiled, wet, or very wrinkled. Check the facility's policy about linen changes. (TNA 265–279; LTCA 210–226)

Take note!

- Always wash your hands before handling clean linen and after handling dirty linen.
- Bring enough linen to the person's room. Extra linen in the room is considered contaminated. It is not used for other persons. Put it with the dirty laundry so that it is not used for other persons.
- Linens the person will lie on must be wrinkle-free and tight. The cotton drawsheet must completely cover a plastic drawsheet, if used. Change the linen of incontinent persons promptly.
- Linens that are wet, damp, or soiled must be changed right away.
- Follow the principles of good body mechanics when making beds.
- Make as much of one side of the bed as possible before going to the other side. This saves time and energy.

Skills list

Making an Unoccupied (Open) Bed, page 119
Making an Occupied Bed, page 120

Questions for review (Answers to these questions are on page 92)

Circle the best answer.

1. Mr. Jones is sitting in a chair while his bed is being made. The top linens are folded back so that he can get into bed. This is a(n)
   a. open bed.
   b. closed bed.
   c. surgical bed.
   d. occupied bed.

2. You are removing dirty linen from the bed. You should
   a. roll linen away from you.
   b. shake linens to remove loose particles.
   c. place dirty linen on the floor away from clean linen.
   d. keep linen close to you when removing it from the room.

3. Which of the following statements is **FALSE**?
   a. Place dirty linen in a hamper.
   b. Bottom linens must be wrinkle-free and tight.
   c. Leftover linen can be used for another resident.
   d. Make as much of one side of the bed as possible before going to the other side.

4. You are gathering linen to make a bed. It is best to
   a. collect linen from the top shelves first.
   b. collect linen in the order of placement on the bed.
   c. collect extra linen in case some pieces are dropped.
   d. collect linen in the opposite order of placement on the bed.

5. A resident will be out of bed most of the day. You should make a(n)
   a. open bed.
   b. closed bed.
   c. surgical bed.
   d. occupied bed.

6. Plastic drawsheets do the following **EXCEPT**
   a. protect the mattress.
   b. protect the bottom linens.
   c. increase the resident's comfort.
   d. increase the risk of skin breakdown.

7. When making a bed, the nursing assistant needs to follow the rules of
   a. surgical asepsis.
   b. sterile technique.
   c. medical asepsis.
   d. isolation precautions.

8. You have extra linen in a resident's room. You can
   a. put the linen back onto the linen cart.
   b. use the linen for the resident's roommate.
   c. take the linen to another resident's room to save costs.
   d. put the linens in the dirty laundry since they are contaminated.

9. You are making an occupied bed. To remove bottom linens, you should
   a. tuck the bottom linens under the resident.
   b. roll the linens up from the bottom of the bed.
   c. remove them when the resident gets out of bed.
   d. raise the resident off the bed with a mechanical lift.

10. The following observations are made about a closed bed. Which is **INCORRECT**?
    a. The top linen is tucked in on the sides.
    b. The top sheet is turned down over the blanket.
    c. The open end of the pillow is away from the door.
    d. The signal light is attached on top of the bed within resident reach.

Chapter 7   *Cleanliness and skin care*

WORDS TO REMEMBER

alopecia   Hair loss; hair loss may be complete or partial

AM care   Routine care performed before breakfast; early morning care

aspiration   Breathing fluid or an object into the lungs

bedsore   A pressure sore; a pressure ulcer

dandruff   The excessive amount of dry, white flakes from the scalp

evening care   HS or PM care

friction   The rubbing of one surface against another

HS care   Care given in the evening at bedtime; evening care or PM care

morning care   Care given after breakfast; cleanliness and skin care measures are more thorough at this time

oral hygiene   Measures performed to keep the mouth and teeth clean; mouth care

pericare   Perineal care

perineal care   Cleansing the genital and anal areas

PM care   HS care or evening care

pressure sore   An area where the skin and underlying tissues are eroded because of the lack of blood flow; a bedsore; a pressure ulcer

pressure ulcer   A bedsore; a pressure sore

DAILY CARE OF THE PERSON

Personal hygiene practices are performed as often as needed to keep the person clean and comfort-able. Certain routines are performed at regular intervals each day. Early morning or AM care is performed by night or day shift staff before breakfast is served. Personal hygiene measures performed at this time include:

- Offering a bedpan, urinal, or assisting the person to the bathroom
- Helping the person wash his or her face and hands
- Assisting the person with oral hygiene
- Positioning the person in Fowler's position or in a bedside chair for breakfast
- Straightening the person's bed linens
- Straightening the person's unit

Morning care is given after breakfast. Cleanliness and skin care measures are more thorough at this time. Routine morning care measures usually involve:

- Offering a bedpan or urinal or assisting the person to the bathroom
- Helping the person wash his or her face and hands
- Assisting the person with oral hygiene
- Shaving the person
- Providing a shower, tub bath, or bed bath for the person
- Giving the person perineal care
- Giving the person a back massage
- Changing the person's gown or pajamas, or assisting with dressing
- Brushing or combing the person's hair
- Changing the person's bed linens
- Straightening the person's unit

Afternoon or PM care is performed after lunch and supper. This includes:

- Offering a bedpan or urinal or assisting the person to the bathroom
- Helping the person wash his or her face and hands

- Assisting the person with oral hygiene
- Changing the person's gown, pajamas, or clothing, if needed
- Brushing or combing the person's hair, if needed
- Changing the person's damp or soiled bed linens
- Straightening the person's unit

HS care is given to the person's at bedtime to help promote comfort and relaxation. It involves:

- Offering a bedpan or urinal or assisting the person to the bathroom
- Helping the person wash his or her face and hands
- Assisting the person with oral hygiene
- Changing the person's damp or soiled bed linens and straightening all other bed linens
- Changing the person's gown or pajamas, if needed
- Helping the person who is wearing street clothes to undress and put on a gown or pajamas
- Giving the person a back massage
- Straightening the person's unit (TNA 283–285; LTCA 230–282)

ORAL HYGIENE

Oral hygiene (mouth care) keeps the mouth and teeth clean. It includes care of the teeth, gums, tongue, and mouth. This prevents mouth odors and infections, increases comfort, and makes food taste better. Illness and disease may cause a bad taste in the mouth. Some drugs and diseases cause a coating of the mouth and tongue with a whitish material. Other drugs and diseases cause redness and swelling of the mouth and tongue. A dry mouth is common from some medications, supplemental oxygen, smoking, decreased fluid intake, and anxiety. The nurse assesses the person's need for mouth care and the amount of assistance needed.

When performing or assisting with oral hygiene, the following observations are reported to the nurse:

- Dry, cracked, swollen, or blistered lips
- Redness, swelling, irritation, sores, or white patches in the mouth or on the tongue
- Bleeding, swelling, or redness of the gums (TNA 285–290; LTCA 231–235)

Unconscious persons need special mouth care. Since unconscious persons usually cannot swallow, they must be protected from choking and aspiration. To prevent aspiration, position the person on one side with the head turned well to the side. In this position, excess fluid runs out of the mouth. Thus the risk of aspiration is reduced.

Unconscious persons cannot speak or respond to what is happening. Always assume that unconscious persons can hear. Explain what you are doing step by step. Also tell the person when you are done and when you are leaving the room. (TNA 290–292; LTCA 236–237)

Dentures are cleaned for persons who cannot do so themselves. Mouth care is given and dentures are cleaned as often as natural teeth. Remember, dentures are the person's property and are expensive. Losing or damaging dentures is negligent conduct. When cleaning dentures, hold them firmly over a basin of water lined with a towel. They can easily break or chip if dropped onto a hard surface. Do not use hot water to clean or store dentures. Hot water causes them to warp. If the resident does not wear the dentures, they are stored in a container of cool water. Dentures can dry out and warp if not stored in water.

Dentures are usually removed at bedtime. Remind persons not to wrap dentures in tissues or napkins. There is a risk that they will be discarded. (TNA 292–294; LTCA 238–239)

Take note!

- Oral hygiene is provided on awakening, after each meal, and at bedtime.
- Gloves are worn when providing oral hygiene.
- Let the person perform oral hygiene. Assist as needed.
- Prevent choking by having the person sit up during oral hygiene. If the person cannot sit up, position the person on his or her side. Be sure the person's head is well turned to the side. Mouth care on an unconscious person is usually given at least every 2 hours.
- Dentures are stored in water when not being worn.
- Use soft- or medium-bristled toothbrushes. Clean dentures with a denture cleaner or toothpaste. Glycerin swabs are used for an unconscious person or a person with a sore or tender mouth.
- Use gentle strokes when brushing or flossing the person's teeth.
- Brush all surfaces of the person's teeth, gums, and tongue.
- Inspect the person's mouth, gums, and tongue for:
  a. Dry, cracked, swollen, or blistered lips
  b. Redness, swelling, irritation, sores, or white patches in the mouth or on the tongue
  c. Bleeding, swelling, or excessive redness of the gums
  d. Loose or broken teeth
- Apply petrolatum jelly or other lubricant to chapped, dry, or cracked lips as directed by your supervisor.

Skills list

Brushing the Resident's Teeth, page 122
Denture Care, page 142

Questions for review (Answers to these questions
are on page 93)

Circle the best answer.

1. Which is **NOT** used for oral hygiene?
   a. Toothpaste
   b. Mouthwash
   c. Dental floss
   d. A hard-bristled toothbrush
2. While assisting with oral hygiene, which observation does **NOT** need to be reported?
   a. Pink tongue
   b. Cracked lips
   c. Swollen gums
   d. Bleeding gums
3. For mouth care, the unconscious resident
   should be in
   a. the prone position.
   b. a position of comfort.
   c. the side-lying position.
   d. the Fowler's or semi-Fowler's position.
4. To keep an unconscious resident's mouth open
   during mouth care, you should
   a. use your fingers.
   b. use a washcloth.
   c. use a padded tongue blade.
   d. place toothettes or applicators between the
      teeth.
5. Mouth care is done for all of the following except one. Which is **FALSE**?
   a. To dry the mouth
   b. Prevent infections
   c. Prevent mouth odors
   d. To make food taste better
6. Unconscious residents usually have mouth care
   done
   a. every 2 hours.
   b. every 8 hours.
   c. every 12 hours.
   d. once a day.
7. Flossing is done to remove food between the
   teeth. It is important to
   a. floss more than once a day.
   b. floss between the front teeth only.
   c. allow the floss to go below the gums.
   d. avoid rinsing the mouth after flossing.
8. When cleaning dentures, you should hold them
   a. firmly in both hands.
   b. over an emesis basin.
   c. over a sink full of water.
   d. over a basin of water lined with a towel.
9. Dentures should be cleaned with
   a. soap and hot water.
   b. antiseptic mouthwash.
   c. cold water and dental floss.
   d. toothpaste or denture cleaner.
10. Mouth care for the unconscious resident re-
    quires special precautions. You must prevent
    the resident from
    a. choking on fluids.
    b. eating toothpaste.
    c. talking during the procedure.
    d. biting down on the toothbrush.

BATHING

Bathing cleans the skin and mucous membranes of
the genital and anal areas by removing microorganisms, dead skin, perspiration, and excess oils. A
bath is also refreshing and relaxing. Circulation is
stimulated and body parts are exercised. The bath
provides you an opportunity to make observations
as well as time to talk with and get to know the
person.

Personal choice, weather, physical activity, and
illness affect how often a person bathes. Age also
affects bathing frequency. Dry skin occurs with
aging. Therefore the elderly usually need a complete bath once a week. Partial baths are taken the
other days.

When bathing a person or assisting a person to
bathe, the skin is observed. The following observations are reported to the nurse:

- The color of the skin, lips, nail beds, and sclera
  (whites of the eyes)
- The location and description of rashes
- Dry skin
- Bruises or open skin areas
- Pale or reddened areas, particularly over bony
  parts
- Drainage or bleeding from wounds or body
  openings
- Skin temperature
- Complaints of pain or discomfort

The complete bed bath involves washing the person's entire body in bed. Complete bed baths are
given to persons who cannot bathe themselves. Ask
the nurse about the person's ability to assist with
the bath and any activity or position limits. Many
people have never had a bed bath and may be embarrassed. The person may fear being exposed.
Every person must be given an explanation about
how a bed bath is given and how the body is covered to protect privacy.

The partial bath involves bathing the face,
hands, axillae (underarms), genital and rectal areas,
back, and buttocks. Partial bed baths are given to
persons who cannot bathe themselves. Persons
who are able may bathe themselves in bed or at the
bathroom sink. Nursing personnel assist as needed,
especially with washing the back.

The tub bath is relaxing to many people. A bath lasts no longer than 20 minutes. Safety issues involved with the tub bath include:

- Protecting the person from falling when getting in and out of the tub
- Protecting the person from burns caused by hot water temperatures
- Assessing the person for signs of feeling faint, weak, or tired

Safety measures to prevent falls include:

- Placing a bath mat on the bottom of the tub, unless there are nonskid strips or a nonskid surface
- Placing needed items within the person's reach (including the call bell)
- Draining the tub before the person gets out of the tub; keep the person covered to protect from exposure and chilling
- Directing the person to use safety bars when getting in and out of the tub
- Avoiding the use of bath oils; they make tub surfaces slippery

A shower may be part of the bathtub or a separate stall. A weak or paralyzed person can use a shower chair. The shower chair is wheeled into the shower stall. Shower chairs are made of plastic, with wheels on the legs. Water drains through a round, open area in the seat. The wheels are locked during the shower to prevent the chair from moving. Persons must be protected from falling and chilling. Privacy is also protected. Do not leave someone unattended in the shower. (TNA 295–305; LTCA 240–253)

Perineal Care

Perineal care is done at least once a day during the bath. The procedure is also done when the area is contaminated with urine and feces. Persons should do their own perineal care, if able. The person should be allowed to do perineal care without assistance, if able. Otherwise it is done by a member of the nursing team. Care must always be taken to maintain privacy and avoid embarrassing the person.

Gloves are required for perineal care. Work from the cleanest area to the dirtiest. The urethral area is the cleanest and the anal area the dirtiest. Therefore clean from the urethra to the anal area. The perineal area is very delicate and easily injured. Use warm water, not hot. The area must be rinsed thoroughly. Pat dry after rinsing to reduce moisture and promote comfort. (TNA 308–311; LTCA 256–259)

Perineal care is given to the female by separating the labia with one hand. Use a mitted washcloth to cleanse between the labia with downward strokes. The rectal area is cleaned by wiping from the vagina to the anus. The side-lying position allows the anal area to be cleaned more thoroughly.

The foreskin of the uncircumcised male is pulled back for perineal care. It is returned to the normal position immediately after cleaning. The penis is cleaned with circular motions starting at the urethra. (TNA 308–311; LTCA 256–259)

Take note!

- A person may get a complete or partial bed bath, a tub bath, or a shower.
- The person should be given choices with regard to the time of day and frequency of receiving a bath.
- Consult the nursing care plan about the type of bath a person should have .
- Skin care products cleanse, protect, lubricate, absorb moisture, and help with body odors. Find out which skin care products to use during the bath. Allow personal choice when possible.
- Protect the person's privacy during the bath. Properly screen the person and close doors.
- During the bed bath, make sure the person is well covered for warmth and privacy.
- The water temperature should be:
  a. 110° to 115° F (43° to 46° C) for a complete bed bath and a partial bath
  b. 105° F (41° C) for a tub bath
  c. 105° to 109° F (41° to 43° C) for perineal care
- Keep soap in the soap dish between latherings. This prevents the water from becoming very soapy. If a tub bath or shower is taken, the person will not slip on the soap.
- Make a mitt with the washcloth. Use a mitt throughout the procedure.
- Wash from the cleanest to the dirtiest areas.
- Rinse the skin thoroughly to remove all soap.
- Pat the skin dry to avoid irritating or breaking the skin.
- Bathe the skin whenever fecal material or urine is on the skin.
- Follow universal precautions when giving a bath.
- The tub is cleaned before use to prevent the spread of microbes and infection.

Skills list

Questions for review (Answers to these questions are on page 93)

Circle the best answer.

1. The best time to bathe a resident is
   a. after breakfast.
   b. before lunch.

c. before bedtime.

d. at the time preferred by the resident.

2. You are to give a partial bath. Which body parts are **NOT** bathed?

a. Genital area

b. Legs and feet

c. Face and hands

d. Back and buttocks

3. Which skin care product protects the skin from the drying effect of air and evaporation?

a. Soap

b. Powder

c. Deodorant

d. Cream or lotion

4. Which statement about bathing is **CORRECT**?

a. Soap is used for all baths.

b. Bathe the dirtiest areas first.

c. You decide the method of bathing a resident.

d. Residents must be protected from drafts and exposure.

5. The purpose of HS care is to

a. increase circulation.

b. prevent body and breath odors.

c. promote cleanliness and skin care.

d. increase comfort and to relax the resident.

6. Water for a bed bath should be between

a. 90° to 100° F.

b. 100° to 105° F.

c. 105° to 110° F.

d. 110° to 115° F.

7. Which of the following actions used when bathing a resident is **FALSE**?

a. Pat the skin dry.

b. Wash from the dirtiest to the cleanest areas.

c. Rinse the skin thoroughly to remove all soap.

d. Cover the resident to provide warmth and privacy.

8. You are to take a resident for a shower. You must protect the resident from

a. falling.

b. fainting.

c. infection.

d. aspiration.

9. An ambulatory resident is taking a tub bath. She should not be in the tub over

a. 5 minutes.

b. 10 minutes.

c. 20 minutes.

d. 30 minutes.

10. A resident is weak and unsteady. To give him a shower, use a

a. bath mat.

b. wheelchair.

c. shower chair.

d. mechanical lift.

11. You are giving a complete bed bath. Which is the correct order for washing body parts?

a. Face, near arm, far arm, and chest

b. Face, far arm, near arm, and chest

c. Near arm, near leg, face, and chest

d. Face, far arm, chest, and near arm

12. You are to give pericare. You will clean from the

a. buttocks to urethra.

b. urethra to the anal area.

c. anal area to the urethra.

d. anal area to the buttocks.

13. Which statement about male perineal care is **TRUE**?

a. Clean the tip of the penis using a circular motion.

b. Clean the shaft of the penis with upward strokes.

c. The anal area is not included in male perineal care.

d. Do not retract the foreskin in uncircumcised residents.

14. Which statement about female perineal care is **FALSE**?

a. Wear disposable gloves.

b. Use warm, not hot water.

c. Wash the anal area using circular motions.

d. Use a washcloth with soap, and clean downward from front to back in one stroke.

15. Why should residents be encouraged to perform perineal care themselves?

a. Residents need to become dependent.

b. Residents will perform pericare more frequently.

c. It is embarrassing to have another wash the perineal area.

d. Residents can clean the area better than the nursing staff.

16. A resident is using a shower chair. The wheels should be

a. locked.

b. unlocked.

c. covered with plastic.

d. removed so they do not get wet and rust.

17. You are giving a resident a bath and notice a reddened area on the resident's heels. You should

a. report your observations to the nurse.

b. rub the area vigorously with the lotion.

c. remember to check the area tomorrow.

d. place a sheepskin under the resident's legs.

18. The best way to use a washcloth for a bed bath is by

a. forming a mitt.

b. folding it in fourths.

c. rolling it securely and holding it like a ball.

d. grasping the cloth loosely and using it like a sponge.

19. When giving a resident a bed bath, which is **INCORRECT**?

a. The room door and windows are closed.

    b. The resident is covered with a bath blanket.
    c. The resident is allowed to wash the genital area.
    d. The bath water is changed once during the bath.
20. A resident has dry, fragile skin. It is important to
    a. bathe the resident daily.
    b. avoid all soaps when bathing.
    c. pat the skin dry and apply lotion.
    d. use water below 100° F for the bath.

DRESSING AND GROOMING

Nursing facility residents often wear street clothes during the day. By wearing a coordinated outfit he or she has personally chosen, the person's body image and sense of self-esteem are improved.

The gown or clothing is changed after the bath and when soiled or wet. Persons who wear regular clothing during the day change into a gown or pajamas for bed. Persons may need help with these activities. Special measures are needed for arm injuries, paralysis, or IV infusions.

A garment that opens in back is removed from the person in the side-lying position. The far side of the garment is tucked under the person. The near side is folded onto the person's chest.

A front-opening garment is removed with the person's head and shoulders raised. The garment is removed from the strong side first. Then it is brought around the back to the weak side. The side-lying position can be used to put on garments that open in the back. The person is turned toward the nursing assistant after the garment is put on the arms. The side of the garment is brought to the person's back. The person is then turned away from the nursing assistant. The other side of the garment is brought to the back and fastened.

A pullover garment is removed from the strong side first. Then the garment is brought up to the person's neck so that it can be removed from the weak side.

Trousers or slacks can be changed with the person in the supine or side-lying position. If the person is in the supine position, the pants can be removed by having the person lift the hips and buttocks. The pants are then slid down over the hips and buttocks. Another way to remove pants is to have the person in the side-lying position. The pants are removed from the strong side first and are slid over the hips and buttocks. The person is turned onto the other side and the pants are removed from the weak side. (TNA 330–340; LTCA 268–275)

Brushing and combing hair is part of the daily care. Encourage persons to do their own hair care. Hair care is performed for those who cannot do so.

Let the person choose how hair is to be brushed, combed, and styled. Brushing and combing keep hair from tangling and matting. When brushing and combing hair, start at the scalp. Then brush or comb to the hair ends. If the hair is matted or tangled, take a small section of hair near the ends and comb or brush through to the hair ends. Working up the scalp, small sections of hair are added. Comb or brush through each longer section to the hair ends. Finally, brush or comb from the scalp to the hair ends.

Long hair is easily matted and tangled. Daily brushing and combing helps prevent the problem. Long hair can be braided (with the person's permission) to help prevent matting and tangling. Special measures are needed for curly, coarse, or dry hair. The person may have certain practices or use special hair products. When planning for hair care, ask the person about personal preferences and hair care measures. (TNA 322–323; LTCA 260–261)

Many factors affect the frequency for shampooing hair. These include the condition of the hair and scalp, hairstyle, and personal choice. Persons often need help shampooing. Personal choice is followed whenever possible. However, safety is important, and the nurse's approval is needed.

There are many ways to shampoo hair. The method used depends on the person's condition, safety factors, and personal choice. The nurse decides the best method for each person. Some persons are able to sit in front of a sink for shampooing. A stretcher can be positioned in front of the sink for those unable to sit or lean backwards. A rubber or plastic trough or shampoo tray can be used for the person confined to bed. The trough protects the bed and lets water drain into a basin on a chair by the bed. Water is poured over the head with a pitcher. (TNA 324–325; LTCA 262–263)

Shaving promotes comfort and psychological well-being. Persons may prefer electric shavers or razor blades. A safety (blade) shaver requires softening the beard and skin beforehand. The skin is softened by applying a warm washcloth or face towel to the face for a few minutes. Then lather the face with soap and water or a shaving cream. Be careful to avoid cutting and irritating the skin.

Beards and mustaches need daily care. Daily washing and combing are usually enough to keep them clean. Ask the person how he wants his beard or mustache groomed. (TNA 326–327; LTCA 264-265)

Nails and feet require special attention to prevent infection, injury, and odors. The feet must be cleaned thoroughly and dried completely. Nursing assistants are not allowed to cut or trim toenails.

Cleaning and trimming fingernails is easier after they have been soaked. Nail clippers are used to cut fingernails. Use extreme caution when clipping and trimming fingernails to prevent damage to the surrounding tissues. (TNA 328–329; LTCA 266–267)

Wearing makeup can improve a woman's body image and self-esteem. Every woman has her own routine for applying makeup. You may need to assist women with applying makeup. Or you may need to apply makeup for the woman. Ask the woman what cosmetics to use, how she wants them applied, and the order of application. Be sure to give her a mirror so she can see how you are applying the makeup. Also offer to touch up her makeup during the day. (TNA 330)

Take note!

- Provide for privacy. Do not expose the person.
- Encourage the person to do as much as possible.
- Allow the person to choose what to wear.
- Remove clothing from the strong or *good* side first. Support the limb while removing the garment.
- Put clothing on the weak or *affected* limb first.
- Never cut hair to remove matted or tangled hair.
- When giving hair care, place a towel across the shoulders to protect the person's gown or clothing.
- Protect bed linens with a towel when giving hair care in bed.
- Dry and style hair quickly to avoid chilling the resident.
- When using electric shavers, practice safety precautions for electrical equipment.
- Razor blades can cause nicks or cuts. Universal precautions and the Bloodborne Pathogen Standard are followed to prevent contact with the person's blood.
- Shave in the direction of the hair growth. Long strokes are used on the larger areas of the face. Short strokes are used around the chin and lips.
- Apply direct pressure to any nicks or cuts. Report any nicks or cuts to the nurse immediately.
- Never trim or shave a beard or mustache without the person's consent.
- Soak the person's fingernails before trimming.
- Trim the person's fingernails straight across with a clipper.

Skills list

Dressing the Resident, page 144
Brushing and Combing the Resident's Hair, page 146
Giving Nail and Foot Care, page 147

Questions for review (Answers to these questions are on page 94)

Circle the best answer.

1. Which should you do **FIRST** when shaving Mr. Jones?
   a. Wash his face.
   b. Apply a generous amount of lather.
   c. Shave in the direction of the hair growth.
   d. Apply a wet washcloth or towel to his face.
2. A good way to prevent long hair from matting or tangling is to
   a. oil the hair.
   b. cut the hair.
   c. braid the hair.
   d. shampoo the hair.
3. Mrs. Adams has right-sided paralysis. To remove a blouse begin
   a. with the left arm.
   b. with the right arm.
   c. by turning her onto her left side.
   d. by placing the clean garment on the affected arm first.
4. A resident has an IV. When changing the gown, you should
   a. cut the sleeve to remove the arm.
   b. remove the gown from the affected arm first.
   c. remove the gown from the unaffected arm first.
   d. disconnect the tubing from the bottle so you can remove the gown.
5. When brushing the resident's hair
   a. start at the back of the head.
   b. brush from the scalp to the hair ends.
   c. leave the resident's eyeglasses in place.
   d. brush from the nape of the neck upward.
6. You are shampooing a resident's hair in bed. Which is **INCORRECT**?
   a. Work up a lather using both hands.
   b. Massage the scalp with your fingertips.
   c. Water should be approximately 110° F.
   d. Place a washcloth or hand towel over the resident's face.
7. Mrs. Turner asks to have her hair shampooed. You should
   a. report the request to the nurse.
   b. tell the family to call a beautician.
   c. suggest that brushing and combing be done instead.
   d. take the resident to the shampoo sink and set up the equipment.
8. If nicks occur while you are shaving a resident, you should
   a. apply aftershave lotion to the area.
   b. apply direct pressure to the bleeding area.
   c. wait until the bleeding stops to finish shaving.
   d. apply an adhesive bandage to any bleeding area.
9. You are to shampoo a resident's hair in bed. You will need all of the following **EXCEPT**
   a. shampoo.
   b. a water pitcher.

c. hand-held spray nozzle.

d. a rubber or plastic trough.

10. Which statement about nail care is **INCORRECT**?

a. Cut fingernails straight across.

b. Trim toenails after trimming fingernails.

c. Soak nails in warm water before trimming.

d. Do not use scissors when trimming fingernails.

BACK MASSAGE

The back massage (back rub) relaxes muscles and stimulates circulation. The massage is normally given after the bath and with HS care. It should last 3 to 5 minutes. Observe the skin before starting the procedure for breaks in the skin, bruises, reddened areas, and other signs of skin breakdown. Lotion is used to reduce friction when giving the massage. It is warmed before being applied. Check with the nurse before giving back massages to persons with heart, back, skin, or lung conditions. (TNA 306–307; LTCA 254–255)

Take note!

- Warm the lotion by placing the bottle in warm bath water, holding it under warm running water, or holding some lotion in your hands for a short time.
- The prone position is best for the back massage. The side-lying position is also used.
- Use long, firm strokes. Your hands should be in contact with the person's skin at all times.

- Use circular motions with the tips of your index and middle fingers to massage bony areas.
- Use fast movements to stimulate and slow movements to relax the person.

Questions for review (Answers to these questions are on page 95)

Circle the best answer.

1. A back massage is given to

a. relax muscles.

b. contract muscles.

c. decrease circulation.

d. exercise the resident.

2. The back rub should last

a. 1 to 2 minutes.

b. 3 to 5 minutes.

c. 8 to 10 minutes.

d. 12 to 15 minutes.

3. To reduce friction during a back massage use

a. soap.

b. lotion.

c. bath oil.

d. rubbing alcohol.

4. Which position is **BEST** for a back massage?

a. Prone

b. Supine

c. Fowler's

d. Side-lying

5. The back massage should end with

a. fast movements.

b. circular movements.

c. kneading movements.

d. long, firm movements.

Chapter 8   *Elimination*

WORDS TO REMEMBER

anal incontinence The inability to control the passage of feces and gas through the anus

catheter A tube used to drain or inject fluid through a body opening

colostomy An artificial opening between the colon and abdominal wall

constipation The passage of a hard, dry stool

defecation The process of excreting feces from the rectum through the anus; a bowel movement

diarrhea The frequent passage of liquid stools

dysuria Painful or difficult *(dys)* urination *(uria)*

fecal impaction The prolonged retention and accumulation of feces in the rectum

feces The semi-solid mass of waste products in the colon

flatulence The excessive formation of gas in the stomach and intestines

flatus Gas or air in the stomach or intestines

functional incontinence The involuntary, unpredicted passage of urine from the bladder; the person does not have nervous system or urinary system diseases or injuries

glucosuria Sugar *(glucos)* in the urine *(uria)*; glycosuria

glycosuria Sugar *(glycos)* in the urine *(uria)*; glucosuria

hematuria Blood *(hemat)* in the urine *(uria)*

ileostomy An artificial opening between the ileum (small intestine) and the abdominal wall

micturition The process of emptying the bladder; urination or voiding

ostomy The surgical creation of an artificial opening

retention catheter A Foley or indwelling catheter

stoma An opening; see colostomy and ileostomy

stool Feces that have been excreted

urinary frequency Voiding at frequent intervals

urinary incontinence The inability to control the passage of urine from the bladder

urinary urgency The need to void immediately

urination The process of emptying the bladder; micturition or voiding

voiding Urination or micturition

MAINTAINING NORMAL URINATION

Healthy adults excrete about 1000 to 1500 ml (2 to 3 pints) of urine a day. Many factors affect the amount of urine produced. The elderly often have problems with urinary elimination.

Urine should be observed carefully for color, clarity, odor, amount, and presence of particles. Normal urine is pale yellow, straw colored, or amber. It is clear with no particles. A faint odor is normal. Abnormal urine is saved and shown to the nurse. Report any complaints of dysuria, burning, or urgency.

You may need to help maintain normal elimination. Some need help getting to the bathroom. Others use bedpans, fracture pans, urinals, and commodes. (TNA 343–352; LTCA 286–306)

Take note!

- Provide the bedpan, urinal, or commode, or help the person to the bathroom as soon as the request is made. The need to void may be urgent.

- Some persons are too weak, embarrassed, or unable to ask. Offer them the opportunity to void at regular intervals.
- Help the person assume a normal position for voiding, if possible. Women sit or squat; men stand.
- Medical asepsis, universal precautions, and the Bloodborne Pathogen Standard are followed when handling bedpans and their contents.
- Provide fluids as instructed by the nurse.
- Follow the person's normal voiding routines and habits. Check with the nurse and the nursing care plan.
- Cover the person for warmth and privacy.
- Provide for privacy. Pull the curtain around the bed, close doors to the room and bathroom, and pull drapes and window shades. Leave the person alone if permitted.
- Place the call light and toilet paper within reach.
- Tell the person that running water, flushing the toilet, or playing the radio or music can mask urination sounds. This is important for persons embarrassed about voiding with others close by.
- Allow the person enough time to void. Do not rush the person.
- Promote relaxation. Some people like to read when eliminating.
- Run water in a nearby sink if the person has difficulty starting the stream. You may need to place the person's fingers in some water.
- Provide perineal care as needed.
- Let the person wash his or her hands after voiding. Provide a wash basin, soap, washcloth, and towel. Assist as necessary.
- Use fracture pans for persons with limited mobility of the back, and for those with casts, in traction, or who have had hip surgeries.

Skills list

Giving the Bedpan, page 151

Questions for review (Answers to these questions are on page 95)

Circle the best answer.

1. You empty a urinal and observe the following. Which observation needs to be reported?
   a. Urine is clear.
   b. Urine is pale yellow.
   c. Small particles are in the urine.
   d. Urine has a faint ammonia odor.

2. After assisting the resident off the bedpan, what should the nursing assistant do **FIRST**?
   a. Observe the contents.
   b. Empty and rinse the bedpan.
   c. Measure the urine and record the results.
   d. Cover the bedpan and put it in the bathroom.

3. A bedridden female resident has very limited range of motion in her back. Which should she use to urinate?
   a. Urinal
   b. Catheter
   c. Commode
   d. Fracture pan

4. A resident cannot get onto the bedpan. How do you place the bedpan in proper position?
   a. Ask a family member to help you.
   b. Lift the resident's buttocks completely off the mattress.
   c. Turn the resident onto the side near you. Place the bedpan on the far side of the mattress.
   d. Turn the resident onto the side away from you. Place the bedpan firmly against the buttocks.

5. After helping the resident onto the bedpan, commode, or toilet, you should
   a. stand at the bedside.
   b. leave the room and close the door.
   c. sit quietly in a bedside chair and wait.
   d. stay with the resident and straighten up the room.

6. A resident cannot clean the perineal area after urinating. You should
   a. report this to the nurse.
   b. give the resident a partial bath.
   c. clean the perineal area with cotton balls.
   d. clean gently from front to back with toilet tissue.

7. It is best for a man to use the urinal while
   a. sitting.
   b. standing.
   c. lying down.
   d. lying on the left side.

8. Mrs. Smith has used the bedpan. You should do all of the following **EXCEPT**
   a. return the bedpan to the bedside stand.
   b. rinse the bedpan after emptying the urine.
   c. soak the bedpan in disinfectant for 20 minutes.
   d. cover the bedpan and take it to the bathroom or dirty utility room.

9. A commode is
   a. a special urinal.
   b. another name for toilet.
   c. used for residents in traction.
   d. a portable chair with an opening for a bedpan or container.

10. After residents have used the bedpan, urinal, or commode, you should help them to
    a. return to bed.
    b. wash their hands.

c. measure the urine.

d. control urinary elimination.

11. Which of the following observations needs to be reported?

    a. A male resident insists on standing to void.

    b. A resident voids about 30 ml every half hour.

    c. A resident voids about 250 ml every 5 hours.

    d. A resident voids before each meal, at bedtime, and upon awakening.

12. The best position for a woman using the bedpan is

    a. Fowler's position.

    b. The prone position.

    c. The supine position.

    d. The side-lying position.

CATHETERS

An indwelling catheter (retention or Foley catheter) is left in the bladder so urine drains constantly into a drainage bag. A balloon near the tip is inflated after the catheter is inserted to keep the catheter from slipping out of the bladder. Tubing connects the catheter to the collection bag. Catheter insertion (catheterization) is done by a nurse or doctor. (TNA 352–358; LTCA 294–299)

Catheters require special care. The main goal of catheter care is to prevent infection. This includes cleaning the catheter from the meatus down about 4 inches with soap and water. The Centers for Disease Control (CDC) suggest that perineal care be done daily and after bowel movements. Vaginal drainage may also require frequent perineal care. The catheter is secured to the person's thigh to prevent injuring the urethra. (TNA 353–355; LTCA 296)

Bladder training programs are developed for persons with urinary incontinence. Voluntary control of urination is the goal.

There are two basic methods for bladder training. With one, the person uses the toilet, commode, bedpan, or urinal at scheduled intervals. The person is given 15 or 20 minutes to start voiding. The rules for maintaining normal urination are followed. The second method is used for persons with catheters. This may involve clamping the catheter for varying intervals. When the catheter is removed, assist the person with the toilet, commode, bedpan, or urinal every 2 to 4 hours. (TNA 359; LTCA 299)

Take note!

- Follow the rules of medical asepsis, universal precautions, and the Bloodborne Pathogen Standard.
- Urine must always run freely through the catheter and tubing. The person should not lay on the tubing. Do not allow the tubing to kink.

Coil connecting tubing on the bed and secure it to the bottom linen.

- Keep the collection bag below the level of the bladder. This prevents urine from flowing backward into the bladder.
- Never attach the drainage bag to the side rail. The drainage bag would be higher than the bladder when the side rail is raised. Attach the drainage bag to the bed frame.
- Secure the catheter to the inner thigh or secure it to the man's abdomen. This prevents excessive movement of the catheter and reduces friction at the insertion site. Tape or other devices ordered by the nurse are used to secure catheters.
- Check for leaks. Check the site where the catheter connects to the drainage bag. Report any leaks to the nurse immediately.
- Provide catheter care in addition to perineal care as directed according to facility policy.
- Provide perineal care daily and after bowel movements.
- Empty the bag at the end of the shift or when directed to do so by the nurse. Measure and record the amount of urine. Report increases or decreases in the amount of urine.
- Use a separate measuring container for each person to prevent the spread of microbes from one person to another.
- Do not let the drain on the drainage bag touch any surface.
- Report the following to the nurse:

    a. Complaints of pain, burning, the need to urinate, or irritation

    b. Color, clarity, and odor of urine

Skills list

Catheter Care, page 127

Questions for review (Answers to these questions are on page 96)

Circle the best answer.

1. Other terms used for a Foley catheter are

    a. levine catheter and Fowler's catheter.

    b. Clinitest catheter and Testape catheter.

    c. collecting catheter and drainage catheter.

    d. retention catheter and indwelling catheter.

2. A catheter is held in the bladder by

    a. tape.

    b. muscle control.

    c. an inflated balloon at the tip.

    d. proper positioning of the resident.

3. When a resident is in bed, the collection bag should be attached to the

    a. mattress.

    b. side rails.

c. bed frame.

d. resident's leg.

4. The collection bag is usually emptied
   a. daily.
   b. at bedtime.
   c. every 4 hours.
   d. at the end of every shift.

5. A resident has a Foley catheter. Which is **INCORRECT**?
   a. Coil the connecting tubing on the bed.
   b. Secure the catheter to the resident's thigh.
   c. Keep the connecting tubing free of kinks.
   d. Keep the collection bag above the level of the bladder.

6. When performing catheter care, what should you do **FIRST**?
   a. Make sure the catheter is taped securely.
   b. Check for crusts, abnormal drainage, or secretions.
   c. Clean the catheter from the meatus down about 4 inches.
   d. Apply antiseptic solution with an applicator from front to back.

7. You are emptying a urinary drainage bag. Which is **INCORRECT**?
   a. Collect the urine into a graduate.
   b. Disconnect the bag from the tubing.
   c. Observe the urine for abnormalities.
   d. Open the clamp at the bottom of the bag.

8. A bladder training program has started for a resident with a catheter. Which statement is **CORRECT**?
   a. The catheter will be removed by the nurse.
   b. The resident will be taken to the toilet every 4 hours.
   c. The catheter will be clamped for about 1 hour at the beginning.
   d. The catheter will be clamped for 4 hours, then released for 2 hours.

9. The inability to control the passage of urine from the bladder is called
   a. elimination.
   b. catherization.
   c. urinary incontinence.
   d. involuntary urination.

10. When a resident has a Foley catheter, the main goal is to prevent
    a. pain.
    b. bleeding.
    c. infection.
    d. urination.

COLLECTING AND TESTING URINE SPECIMENS

Urine samples are often collected for laboratory study. The urine tests are used by the doctor to make a diagnosis or to evaluate treatment. In order to obtain accurate results, you need to know how to properly collect each type. A routine urine specimen (random or routine urinalysis) is part of many physical exams. It may be collected at any time. A clean-voided urine specimen (midstream or clean-catch specimen) requires cleaning of the perineal area before voiding. The stream is stopped during voiding, the specimen container positioned, and the urine collected. In a 24-hour urine specimen all urine in a 24-hour period is collected. The test begins by having the person void. This urine is discarded. All of the urine for the next 24 hours is collected and kept chilled on ice or refrigerated. In a fresh-fractional urine sample (double-voided specimen) the person is asked to void to empty the bladder. In 30 minutes the person is asked to void again. This "fresh" urine is tested for sugar. The urine of persons with diabetes mellitus may be tested for sugar and acetone. The doctor orders the type and frequency of these tests. Urine may be tested by using Testape, Clinitest, Acetest, or Keto-Diastix.

If the doctor suspects that a person might have kidney stones (calculi), all of the person's urine is strained. A disposable strainer is placed in a clear, plastic graduate. The urine is poured through the strainer. If a stone is found, it is sent to the laboratory for examination. (TNA 359–367; LTCA 300–305)

Take note!

- Wash your hands before and after collecting the specimen.
- Follow the rules of medical asepsis, universal precautions, and the Bloodborne Pathogen Standard.
- Use a clean container for each specimen.
- Use a container appropriate for the specimen.
- Label the container accurately with the requested information—usually the person's full name, room and bed numbers, date, and time the specimen was collected.
- Do not touch the inside of the container or lid.
- Collect the specimen at the time specified.
- Ask the person not to have a bowel movement while the specimen is being collected. The specimen must be free of fecal material.
- Ask the person not to put toilet tissue in the specimen container. The toilet tissue should be placed in the toilet or wastebasket.
- You may need to position and hold the container for the person when obtaining a specimen.
- Take the specimen to the designated storage place. The specimen should be in a plastic bag.

Questions for review (Answers to these questions are on page 96)

Circle the best answer.

1. When collecting a urine specimen, you should
   a. use the appropriate container.
   b. have the laboratory label the specimen.
   c. collect the specimen when it is convenient.
   d. take the specimen to the lab when it is convenient.

2. A double-voided urine specimen is also called a
   a. random urine specimen.
   b. 24-hour urine specimen.
   c. midstream urine specimen.
   d. fresh-fractional urine specimen.

3. To collect a 24-hour urine specimen, you will need
   a. Testape.
   b. a urine strainer.
   c. a bucket with ice.
   d. antiseptic solution.

4. A routine urine specimen can be obtained
   a. at any time.
   b. only when the resident has eaten.
   c. only after cleaning the perineal area.
   d. only before the resident has breakfast.

5. A midstream urine specimen is ordered. The resident must
   a. save all urine for 24 hours.
   b. be NPO before collecting the specimen.
   c. have perineal care before collecting the specimen.
   d. void once, then collect a urine specimen in 30 minutes.

6. A fractional urine specimen involves having the resident urinate twice. This is because you need
   a. a sterile specimen.
   b. a very fresh specimen.
   c. a large amount of urine.
   d. urine that has been in the bladder several hours.

7. A 24-hour urine specimen involves
   a. straining the urine.
   b. having the resident void once in 24 hours.
   c. collecting a routine urine specimen every hour for 24 hours.
   d. collecting all urine voided by a resident during a 24-hour period.

8. When collecting a 24-hour urine specimen, what should you do with the first voiding?
   a. Discard it.
   b. Send it to the lab.
   c. Test it for sugar and ketones.
   d. Place it in the large container used for saving the urine.

9. Which statement about obtaining a urine sample is **INCORRECT**?
   a. Use a clean container for each specimen.
   b. Wipe the inside of the container with a clean towel.
   c. The resident must not place toilet tissue in the specimen container.
   d. Label the container with the resident's name, room number, the date, and time of collection.

10. You find a stone in the resident's urine. You should
    a. take the stone to the nurse.
    b. let the resident keep the stone.
    c. discard the specimen and the stone.
    d. show the stone to your co-workers.

BOWEL ELIMINATION

Bowel elimination involves the excretion of wastes from the gastrointestinal system. The frequency of bowel movements is highly individualized. Most people develop a personal pattern of regularity. When this pattern is disrupted, elimination problems occur. Many factors affect elimination such as diet, illness, activity, and medications.

The stool is observed before disposal. The following information is reported to the nurse:

- Color
- Amount
- Consistency
- Odor
- Shape
- Size
- Frequency of defecation
- Any complaints of pain (TNA 371–372; LTCA 310–311)

Stool specimens are often collected and sent to the laboratory for study. Fecal material can be checked for blood, fat, microorganisms, worms, and other abnormal contents. Make certain the specimen does not contain urine. (TNA 391–394; LTCA 326–327)

An enema is the introduction of fluid into the rectum and lower colon. Enemas are ordered by doctors. They are usually given to remove feces and to relieve constipation, flatulence, or fecal impaction. Enemas may be ordered before some x-rays.

Various enema solutions are available. The solution is ordered according to the person's needs. A tap-water solution is obtained from a faucet. A soapsuds enema (SSE) is prepared by adding 5 ml of liquid soap to 1000 ml of tap water. A saline solution of salt and water is prepared by adding 2 teaspoons of table salt to 1000 ml of tap water. Oil is used for oil-retention enemas. They are given for constipation or fecal impactions. Commercial enemas are often ordered for constipation. (TNA 376–384; LTCA 313–319)

Rectal tubes are inserted 2 to 4 inches into the rectum to relieve flatulence. The rectal tube is removed after 20 to 30 minutes to help prevent rectal irritation. The nurse tells you when to insert the tube and how long to leave it in place. (TNA 385–386; LTCA 320)

Sometimes surgical removal of part of the intestines is necessary. When a person has a colostomy, part of the colon is brought out onto the abdominal wall and a stoma is made. Fecal material and flatus are expelled through the stoma into a colostomy appliance. This is a disposable plastic bag applied over the stoma. It collects feces expelled through the stoma. Many pouches have a drain at the bottom. When soiled, the drain is opened and the pouch emptied. The pouch **is** changed every 3 to 5 days. The pouch has an adhesive backing that is applied to the skin. A belt may be worn to secure the appliance. (TNA 386–388; LTCA 321–323)

An ileostomy is very similar to a colostomy. A part of the small bowel (the ileum) is brought out onto the abdominal wall and a stoma is made. Fecal material from an ileostomy is liquid and drains constantly. This can be very irritating to the skin. An appliance is placed over the stoma. Because of the continuous fecal drainage, the bag is emptied every 4 to 6 hours or when the person voids. Disposable and reusable ileostomy appliances are available. Reusable pouches are washed with soap and water and allowed to dry and air out. To remove an ileostomy pouch, apply a few drops of solvent to the skin around the pouch. The appliance will loosen and can be gently removed. (TNA 388–390; LTCA 324–325)

Take note!

- Respond promptly to the person's request for a bedpan, commode, or help to the bathroom.
- Provide for the person's privacy, warmth, and comfort. Ask visitors to leave the room when a person asks to use the bedpan, commode, **or** toilet.
- Make sure the call light and toilet tissue are within reach. Leave the room if the person can be left alone. Allow enough time for defecation, but do not delay your return. The person **can** become very weak and uncomfortable if on a bedpan or commode too long.
- Provide perineal care as needed. Let persons wash their hands after they have finished.
- Wear gloves to collect stool specimens. Use a tongue blade to take about 2 tablespoons of feces from the bedpan to the specimen container.
- Enema solutions should be 105° F. In general, 750 to 1000 ml of solution is given. Elderly persons may only be able to retain 500 ml. The left Sims' or the left side-lying position is preferred. Hold the enema bag no more than 18

inches above the mattress. Insert the lubricated enema tubing 2 to 4 inches into the rectum.

- Ostomy odors must be prevented. Good hygiene practice is essential. The pouch is emptied or a new one applied when soiling occurs. Avoiding gas-forming foods helps control odors. Special deodorants can be put into the pouch. The nurse tells you which one to use.
- Very careful skin care must be given to the area around a stoma. Clean the skin around the stoma with water. Use soap or other cleansing agents, if ordered. Rinse and pat dry. Apply a skin barrier to prevent feces from coming in contact with the skin. Then apply the ostomy appliance so that it fits securely to prevent leakage.

Questions for review (Answers to these questions are on page 97)

Circle the best answer.

1. Which statement is **TRUE**?
   a. Feces are always hard and dry.
   b. Feces are normally brown in color.
   c. Defecation only occurs after a meal.
   d. It is abnormal to have a bowel movement every day.
2. Diarrhea is the excretion of
   a. hard, dry stools.
   b. soft, formed stools.
   c. watery and unformed stools.
   d. formed stools with much flatulence.
3. Which statement is **FALSE**?
   a. Exercise stimulates peristalsis.
   b. Aging causes peristalsis to increase.
   c. Gas-forming foods stimulate peristalsis.
   d. Illness and medication can affect bowel elimination.
4. Which statement about enemas is **FALSE**?
   a. Enemas are ordered by doctors.
   b. Enemas help clean the bowel before certain x-ray procedures.
   c. An enema is the introduction of fluid into the rectum and lower colon.
   d. An enema is given whenever a resident has difficulty having a bowel movement.
5. You are assigned to the following residents. Their signal lights are on. Which should you answer **FIRST**?
   a. Mrs. Julian who is constipated
   b. Mr. Wilson who has anal incontinence
   c. Mr. Custer who is bothered with flatus
   d. Mr. Richards who has a fecal impaction
6. The opening surgically created between the colon and the abdomen is called a/an
   a. stoma.
   b. ostomy.

c. ileostomy.

d. colostomy.

7. A resident has an ileostomy. Stool consistency will be
   a. liquid.
   b. soft, formed.
   c. dependent upon the age of the resident.
   d. dependent upon the type of food eaten.

8. A rectal tube is inserted
   a. 1 to 2 inches.
   b. 2 to 4 inches.
   c. 4 to 6 inches.
   d. 8 to 10 inches.

9. An enema solution should be
   a. 95° F.
   b. 100° F.
   c. 105° F.
   d. 110° F.

10. You are giving an enema. The enema bag should be raised
    a. 6 inches above the mattress.
    b. 12 inches above the mattress.
    c. 18 inches above the mattress.
    d. 24 inches above the mattress.

11. Which position is the best for the resident receiving an enema?
    a. Supine
    b. Left side-lying
    c. Semi-Fowler's
    d. Right side-lying

12. Rectal tubes are used to relieve
    a. diarrhea.
    b. flatulence.
    c. constipation.
    d. fecal impaction.

13. An oil-retention enema is given
    a. to relieve flatulence.
    b. to cleanse the bowel.
    c. as part of a bowel training program.
    d. to relieve constipation or fecal impaction.

14. What is used to transfer a stool specimen from the bedpan to the specimen container?
    a. A spoon
    b. Applicators
    c. Tongue blades
    d. Alcohol wipes

15. You are to collect a stool specimen. Which is **FALSE**?
    a. The sample may need to be kept warm.
    b. The resident can urinate at the same time.
    c. The rules of medical asepsis must be followed.
    d. About 2 tablespoons of feces are needed for the sample.

16. When a reusable appliance is used for an ileostomy, you should clean the appliance by
    a. sterilizing it in an autoclave.
    b. sending it home with the family.
    c. washing it with soap and cool water.
    d. sending it to the laundry department.

17. Which can be used to clean the skin around a stoma?
    a. Alcohol
    b. Detergent
    c. Soap and water
    d. Hydrogen peroxide

18. Fecal material from an ileostomy drains
    a. constantly.
    b. every 4 to 6 hours.
    c. when the resident urinates.
    d. after the resident eats or drinks.

19. To remove an ileostomy appliance, you need to use
    a. alcohol.
    b. plain water.
    c. Karaya powder.
    d. a prescribed solvent.

20. All of the following measures help to control colostomy odors **EXCEPT** one. Which is **FALSE**?
    a. Good hygiene
    b. Avoiding gas-forming foods
    c. Rinsing the appliance before reuse
    d. Deodorants placed into the appliance

Chapter 9　　Foods and fluids

WORDS TO REMEMBER

anorexia Loss of appetite

dehydration A decrease in the amount of water in body tissues

dysphagia Difficulty or discomfort *(dys)* in swallowing *(phagia)*

edema The swelling of body tissues with water

gastrostomy A surgically created opening *(stomy)* in the stomach *(gastro)* that allows feeding

graduate A calibrated container used to measure fluid

intake The amount of fluid taken in by the body

intravenous therapy Fluid administered through a needle within a vein; IV, IV therapy, and IV infusion

nutrient A substance that is ingested, digested, absorbed, and used by the body

nutrition The many processes involved in the ingestion, digestion, absorption, and use of foods and fluids by the body

output The amount of fluid lost by the body

FOODS AND FLUIDS

Foods and fluids are needed for health and survival. In the past, good nutrition was based on the four basic food groups: milk and dairy products; meats and fish; fruits and vegetables; and breads and cereals. In 1992 the US Dept. of Agriculture (USDA) released its "Food Guide Pyramid" (Fig. 4) to replace the four basic food groups. A well-balanced diet contains foods from the five food groups in levels 1, 2, and 3. The diet provides the necessary amounts of proteins, carbohydrates, fats, vitamins, and minerals.

Protein is the most important nutrient—it is needed for tissue growth and repair. Protein sources include meat, fish, poultry, eggs, milk and milk products, cereals, beans, peas, and nuts.

Carbohydrates provide energy. They also provide fiber for bowel elimination. Carbohydrates are found in fruits, vegetables, breads, cereals, and sugar.

Fats provide energy and serve many other functions. They add flavor to food and help the body use certain vitamins. Fats also conserve body heat and protect organs from injury. Fat sources include the fat in meats, lard, butter, shortenings, salad and vegetable oils, milk, cheese, egg yolks, and nuts.

Although they do not provide calories, vitamins are essential nutrients. They are ingested through food. Vitamins A, D, E, and K can be stored by the body. Vitamin C and the B complex vitamins are not stored. They must be ingested daily. Each vitamin is needed for certain body functions.

A well-balanced diet also supplies needed amounts of minerals. Minerals are used for many body processes. They are needed for bone and tooth formation, nerve and muscle function, fluid balance, and other body processes.

Eating habits vary among individuals and are affected by many factors, including religion and culture. When assisting a person with eating, try to make the meal as pleasant as possible. (TNA 397–407; LTCA 332–338)

Doctors often order special diets for a nutritional deficiency or a disease, to eliminate or decrease certain substances in the diet, or for weight control. For example, a low-cholesterol diet limits intake of fatty foods such as red meat, ice cream, and eggs. Special diets are ordered for persons before and after surgery and for those with diabetes.

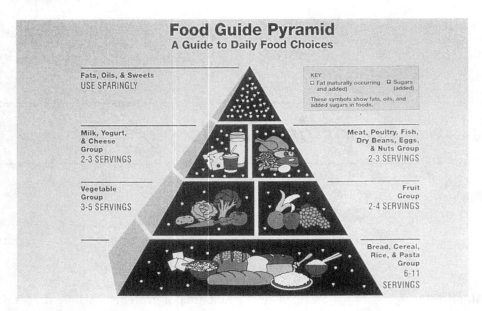

Fig. 4 Food Guide Pyramid. (Courtesy U.S. Dept. of Agriculture; from Sorrentino SA: *Mosby's Textbook for Nursing Assistants,* ed 4, St Louis, 1996, Mosby-Year Book.)

Persons with diseases of the heart, kidneys, gallbladder, liver, stomach, or intestines may receive special diets. Allergies also require special diets. Many persons do not need special diets. Regular diet, general diet, and house diet mean that there are no dietary limits, restrictions, or modifications. The sodium-restricted diet and diabetic diet are often ordered. A diabetic diet is very strict. Meals must be served at regular intervals, the amounts of calories and carbohydrates consumed are important, and all food served must be eaten (and only what is served).

Fluid balance is essential for health and life. The amount of fluid taken into the body must equal the amount lost. Fluid is lost through the urine, feces, skin, and lungs. Doctors and nurses use this information to evaluate a person's fluid balance. You need to keep accurate intake and output records as directed. (TNA 412–415; LTCA 342–345)

In nursing facilities, residents rely on the nursing team to meet part or all of their food and fluid needs. Some residents are in special dining programs. Some need to be fed. Remember that meals provide opportunities for pleasure and socialization. The person will enjoy the meal even more if refreshed and in a comfortable position.

When feeding a person, engage him or her in pleasant conversation. However, give the person enough time to chew and swallow. Also, sit so that you face the person. By facing the person, you can see how well the person is eating. You can also see if the person has problems swallowing. Ask the person about the order in which to offer foods and fluids. Spoons are used to feed the person since they are less likely to cause injury. The spoon should be only one-third full.

Visually impaired persons are often keenly aware of food aromas. Be sure to tell the person what foods and fluids are on the tray. When feeding someone who is visually impaired, always tell the person what you are offering. If the person does not need to be fed, identify the foods and fluids and their location on the tray. Use the numbers on a clock to identify the locations of foods. (TNA 415–418; LTCA 345–348)

Take note!

- Meals in health care facilities are planned to provide balanced nutrition. Encourage persons to eat from all of the food groups served.
- Elderly persons often need special diets. They are ordered because of a nutritional deficiency, disease, or to change the amounts of certain substances in the diet. Make sure that the person receives the correct meal tray.
- Persons must be comfortable and their surroundings free of unpleasant sights, sounds, or odors. Provide oral hygiene, and meet the person's eliminating needs before meals. See that the bedridden person is clean and dry and in a comfortable position.
- Serve meals promptly. Assist with meals as needed. Encourage persons to feed themselves as much as possible. Be supportive and patient.
- Fresh drinking water should be given to each person. Some may have fluid restrictions. Check with the nurse.
- Between-meal nourishments are part of therapeutic diet plans. They must be served on time.
- Keep accurate records when a person is placed on intake and output (I&O). Measure fluids with a graduate and record in milliliters (ml) or in cubic centimeters (cc). The person

or family can participate if correctly shown how to record intake. Remind the person to use the urinal, commode, bedpan, or specimen pan for urination.

Skills list

Feeding the Resident, page 130
Measuring Intake and Output, page 129

Questions for review (Answers to these questions are on page 98)

Circle the best answer.

1. Milk and dairy products are **NOT** high in
   a. fat.
   b. protein.
   c. calcium.
   d. vitamins A and C.
2. How many servings of bread do normal adults need daily?
   a. 2
   b. 4
   c. 6
   d. 15
3. A good source of vitamin C is
   a. liver.
   b. oranges.
   c. sunlight.
   d. fish liver oils.
4. Which statement about vitamins is **FALSE**?
   a. They are ingested through food.
   b. They cannot be stored in the body.
   c. They do not provide any calories.
   d. They are not produced by the body.
5. A serving of meat or fish is considered to be
   a. 2 to 3 ounces.
   b. 4 to 6 ounces.
   c. 8 ounces.
   d. 12 ounces or more.
6. Between-meal nourishments are served
   a. after meals.
   b. when it is convenient to do so.
   c. when fresh drinking water is served.
   d. when they arrive on the nursing unit.
7. Edema means
   a. increased appetite.
   b. decreased appetite.
   c. body tissues are swollen with water.
   d. there is a decreased amount of water in body tissues.
8. When feeding residents, offer food
   a. in a clockwise fashion.
   b. as you would eat the food.
   c. as preferred by the resident.
   d. in a counterclockwise fashion.
9. A resident is blind. Identify the location of the food on the tray by
   a. using numbers of a clock.
   b. letting the resident smell each food.
   c. giving the resident a taste of each item.
   d. guiding the resident's hand to each item and saying what it is.
10. Which resident should **NOT** receive fresh drinking water?
    a. A blind resident
    b. The resident who is NPO
    c. The resident who is on a general diet
    d. The resident who has a force fluid order
11. Measure output by using a/an
    a. graduate.
    b. emesis basin.
    c. water pitcher.
    d. measuring cup.
12. Which statement about diabetic diets is **FALSE**?
    a. Meals must be served at regular intervals.
    b. Calories are not a concern in the diabetic diet.
    c. The amount of carbohydrates in the diet is controlled.
    d. The resident must eat only what is allowed and all that is allowed.
13. Which is **NOT** allowed on a low-cholesterol diet?
    a. Bread
    b. Potatoes
    c. Ice cream
    d. Skimmed milk
14. Which is **NOT** important before serving a meal to a resident?
    a. Change the resident's gown.
    b. Assist the resident with oral hygiene.
    c. Assist the resident into a comfortable position.
    d. Offer the bedpan or urinal or assist the resident to the bathroom.
15. For normal fluid balance, adults require
    a. 1000 to 1500 ml daily.
    b. 1500 to 2000 ml daily.
    c. 2000 to 2500 ml daily.
    d. 2500 to 3000 ml daily.
16. Which of the following are **NOT** recorded as intake?
    a. Coffee, tea, juices, and soft drink
    b. Butter, sauces, and melted cheese
    c. Jello, popsicles, and creamed cereals
    d. Ice cream, sherbert, custard, and pudding

17. How many milliliters are in this graduate (Fig. 5)?
   a. 5
   b. 11
   c. 150
   d. 350

18. How many cubic centimeters (cc) are in this graduate (Fig. 6)?
   a. 10
   b. 150
   c. 300
   d. 350

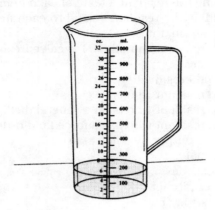

Fig. 5

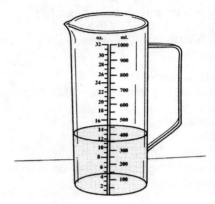

Fig. 6

Chapter 10   *Vital signs*

WORDS TO REMEMBER

apical-radial pulse Taking the apical and radial pulses at the same time; these rates should be equal.

apnea The lack or absence of *(a)* breathing *(pnea)*

blood pressure The amount of force exerted against the walls of an artery by the blood

bradypnea Slow *(brady)* breathing *(pnea)*; the respiratory rate is less than 10 respirations per minute

diastolic pressure The pressure in the arteries when the heart is at rest

dyspnea Difficult, labored, or painful *(dys)* breathing *(pnea)*

pulse The beat of the heart felt at an artery as a wave of blood passes through the artery

pulse deficit The difference between the apical and radial pulse rates; it is found by subtracting the radial from the apical rate

pulse rate The number of heartbeats or pulses felt in 1 minute

respiration The act of breathing air into (inhalation) and out of (exhalation) the lungs

sphygmomanometer The instrument used to measure blood pressure

stethoscope An instrument used to listen to the sounds produced by the heart, lungs, and other body organs

systolic pressure The amount of force it takes to pump blood out of the heart into the arterial circulation

tachypnea Rapid *(tachy)* breathing *(pnea)*; the respiratory rate is usually greater than 24 respirations per minute

vital signs Temperature, pulse, respirations, and blood pressure

MEASUREMENT OF VITAL SIGNS

The vital signs reflect the function of three life processes: breathing, heart function, and regulation of body temperature. Vital signs detect changes in normal body function and determine a person's response to treatment. Many factors affect vital signs. They include sleep, activity, eating, weather, noise, exercise, medications, fear, anxiety, and illness. (TNA 427; LTCA 358)

The nurse tells you when to obtain vital signs. They must be measured accurately and reported promptly.

Body temperature is the amount of heat in the body. Body temperature rises slightly with meals and daily activity. Thermometers are used to measure temperature. Glass, electronic, tympanic membrane, disposable, and temperature-sensitive tape thermometers are available. The Fahrenheit (F) and Centigrade or Celsius (C) scales are used to measure temperature. Common sites for measuring body temperature are the mouth, rectum, axilla (underarm), and ear (tympanic). Normal body temperature depends on the site:

- Oral: 98.6° F (37° C)
- Rectal: 99.6° F (37.5° C)
- Axillary: 97.6° F (36.5° C)
- Tympanic: 98.6° F (37° C)

(TNA 428–440; LTCA 358–371)

The pulse can be felt in a number of places (Fig. 7). The radial site is used the most. The apical

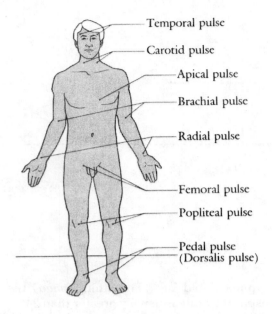

Temporal pulse

Carotid pulse

Apical pulse

Brachial pulse

Radial pulse

Femoral pulse

Popliteal pulse

Pedal pulse
(Dorsalis pulse)

Fig. 7 Pulse sites. (From Sorrentino SA: *Mosby's Textbook for Nursing Assistants,* ed 4, St Louis, 1996, Mosby-Year Book.)

pulse is felt over the apex of the heart. Apical pulses are taken on persons who have heart diseases or who are taking medications that affect the heart. The apical pulse is taken with a stethoscope. The adult pulse rate is between 60 and 100 beats per minute. A rate of less than 60 or greater than 100 is considered abnormal. Abnormal rates are reported to the nurse immediately. (TNA 440–447; LTCA 371–377)

Each respiration is one inhalation and one exhalation. The chest rises as oxygen is taken into the lungs (inhalation) and falls as carbon dioxide is moved out of the lungs (exhalation). Breathing is under voluntary control. Therefore the person should not be aware that the respiratory rate is being counted. Normal respirations occur between 10 and 20 times per minute in the adult. Many abnormal breathing patterns can be seen. (TNA 448; LTCA 378)

Blood pressure measures both the systolic and diastolic pressures. The period of heart muscle contraction is called systole. The period of heart muscle relaxation is called diastole. Both the systolic and diastolic pressures are measured. The average adult has a systolic pressure of 120 mm Hg and a diastolic pressure of 80 mm Hg. This is written as 120/80 mm Hg. A stethoscope and sphygmomanometer are used to measure blood pressure. (TNA 450–453; LTCA 379–381)

Take note!

- The normal ranges of body temperature for adults are:

  Oral—97.6° to 99.6° F (36.5° to 37.5° C)
  Rectal—98.6° to 100.6° F (37.0° to 38.1° C)
  Axillary—96.6° to 98.6° F (36.0° to 37.0° C)
  Ear—98.6° F (37° C)

- Shake down a glass thermometer before taking a temperature. This moves the mercury into the bulb. Check for breaks or chips that could cause injury.

- A glass thermometer needs to remain in place for 2 to 3 minutes for an accurate measurement. Electronic thermometers measure temperature in 2 to 60 seconds. Tympanic thermometers measure temperature in 1 to 3 seconds. Disposable oral thermometers require 45 to 60 seconds. Temperature-sensitive tape changes color in response to body heat in about 15 seconds.

- Rectal temperatures are taken on some people. This includes those who are receiving oxygen, confused, disoriented, restless, or delirious. The rectal thermometer is lubricated and inserted into the anal opening about 1 inch. Glass thermometers are held in place for at least 2 minutes. Less time is needed for electronic devices.

- Axillary temperatures are the least accurate. The axilla must be dry. The thermometer is held in place 5 to 10 minutes.

- Stethoscopes are often shared among workers. Clean the earpieces and diaphragm before and after each use. Cleaning prevents the spread of microorganisms.

- The normal adult pulse rate ranges between 60 and 100 beats per minute. The rhythm and force or strength of the pulse also must be assessed.

- The pulse is felt by placing the first three fingers of one hand against the radial artery. Do not use your thumb to take a pulse since the thumb has a pulse of its own. The pulse is counted for 30 seconds. That number is multiplied by two for the number of beats per minute. Irregular pulses are counted for a full minute. Some facilities require that all pulses be taken for 1 full minute. You need to follow your facility's policy.

- The apical pulse is located on the left side of the chest slightly below the nipple. The pulse is counted for a full minute using a stethoscope. The "lub-dub" sound is counted as one beat.

- An apical-radial pulse is taken by two workers at the same time. One person counts the radial pulse; the other counts the apical pulse. The rates should be equal. If not, the difference is recorded as the pulse deficit.

- Respirations are counted right after the pulse. The person assumes the pulse is still being taken. Respirations are counted by watching the rise and fall of the chest for 30 seconds. Multiply that number by two. If the breathing is abnormal, count respirations for a full minute.

- Many factors can affect blood pressure. Normal adult ranges are: systolic pressure between 100 and 140 mm Hg; diastolic pressure between 60 and 90 mm Hg. In the elderly, the blood pressure may be higher but still normal. A systolic pressure between 100 and 160 mm Hg and a diastolic pressure between 60 and 95 mm Hg is normal for the elderly. When the systolic and diastolic pressures are consistently above normal, the condition is called hypertension.

- Systolic pressures below 90 mm Hg and diastolic pressures below 60 mm Hg are called hypotension. Some people normally have low blood pressures. However, hypotension is a sign of a serious condition that can lead to death if not corrected.

- Blood pressures should not be measured on an arm with an IV, a cast, or an injury. If the resident has had breast surgery, do not measure a blood pressure in the arm on the affected side.

- Allow the resident to rest about 15 minutes before measuring the blood pressure. Place the cuff around the bare upper arm at least 1 inch above the elbow.

- Place the stethoscope earpieces in your ears and place the diaphragm of the stethoscope firmly over the brachial artery. Inflate the cuff 30 mm Hg beyond the point at which you last felt the pulse.

- Deflate the cuff at an even rate of 2 to 4 millimeters per second.

- Note the point on the scale where you hear the first sound. This is the systolic reading. It should be near the point where the radial pulse disappeared.

- Continue to deflate the cuff. Note the point where the sound disappears for the diastolic reading.

Skills list

Measuring the Oral Temperature, page 131
Measuring Pulse, page 132
Measuring Respirations, page 133
Measuring Blood Pressure, page 134

Questions for review (Answers to these questions are on page 98)

Circle the best answer.

1. Which body process is **NOT** measured by vital signs?
   a. Respirations
   b. Heart function
   c. Bowel function
   d. Body temperature

2. A sphygmomanometer is used to measure
   a. pulse rate.
   b. respirations.
   c. blood pressure.
   d. body temperature.

3. Body temperature is usually lowest
   a. after a meal.
   b. in the afternoon.
   c. late in the evening.
   d. in the early morning.

4. Which temperature should be reported immediately?
   a. 97.6° F axillary
   b. 99.0° F orally
   c. 99.2° F rectally
   d. 102.4° F orally

5. You are to take a rectal temperature with a glass thermometer. Which is **INCORRECT**?
   a. Hold the thermometer in place for 2 minutes.
   b. Lubricate the end of the thermometer before insertion.
   c. Insert the thermometer about 6 inches into the rectum.
   d. Shake down the thermometer until the mercury is below the lines and numbers.

6. To clean a glass thermometer, you should
   a. wipe the thermometer with alcohol.
   b. wipe the thermometer with a tissue.
   c. wash the thermometer in hot, soapy water.
   d. wash the thermometer in cold, soapy water.

7. An oral temperature taken with an electronic thermometer requires
   a. less than 1 minute.
   b. 1 to 2 minutes.
   c. 3 to 4 minutes.
   d. 8 to 11 minutes.

8. Which axillary temperature is abnormal?
   a. 36° C
   b. 96.6° F
   c. 98.6° F
   d. 99.6° F

9. An oral temperature should **NOT** be taken if a resident
   a. has diarrhea.
   b. is receiving oxygen.
   c. has heart disease.
   d. is alert and cooperative.

10. For an oral temperature, the thermometer is placed
    a. under the tongue.
    b. next to the cheek.
    c. between the teeth.
    d. on top of the tongue.

11. Which of the following pulses should be reported immediately?

a. A resident has a pulse of 62 beats per minute.
b. A resident has a pulse of 72 beats per minute.
c. A resident has a pulse of 80 beats per minute.
d. A resident has a pulse of 120 beats per minute.

12. Which site is usually used to take a pulse?
    a. The apical pulse
    b. The radial pulse
    c. The brachial pulse
    d. The femoral pulse

13. Which statement about taking a pulse is **TRUE**?
    a. The pulse can be taken with any of the fingers.
    b. The pulse is normally thready and hard to find.
    c. An irregular pulse must be taken for one full minute.
    d. The pulse is taken for 15 seconds and multiplied by four.

14. A resident's pulse is very difficult to feel. Report that the pulse is
    a. regular.
    b. irregular.
    c. full and bounding.
    d. weak and thready.

15. Before using a stethoscope, you should
    a. replace the earpiece.
    b. wash it in soap and water.
    c. make sure it has been sterilized.
    d. wipe the earpieces and diaphragm with alcohol.

16. An apical pulse is counted for
    a. 1 full minute.
    b. 30 seconds, then multiplied by 2.
    c. 15 seconds, then multiplied by 4.
    d. as long as it takes to hear a regular beat.

17. The apical pulse is located
    a. on the thumb side of the wrist.
    b. just above the bend in the elbow on the inside of the arm.
    c. 2 to 3 inches to the left of the breastbone and below the left nipple.
    d. 2 to 3 inches to the right of the breastbone and below the right nipple.

18. You are taking a resident's respirations. Which is **INCORRECT**?
    a. Watch the rise and fall of the resident's chest.
    b. Hold the resident's wrist as if you are counting the pulse.
    c. Count the respirations for 30 seconds and multiply by 2.
    d. Tell the resident you are going to count how many times he breathes.

19. Tachypnea means that respirations are
    a. normal.
    b. labored and difficult.
    c. less than 10 per minute.
    d. greater than 24 per minute.

20. Apnea is
    a. rapid breathing.
    b. the absence of breathing.
    c. slow, shallow, and irregular breathing.
    d. rapid and deeper than normal breathing.

21. Which blood pressure reading is abnormal?
    a. 120/70 mm Hg
    b. 130/70 mm Hg
    c. 140/90 mm Hg
    d. 180/100 mm Hg

22. Which artery is normally used to measure a blood pressure?
    a. Carotid
    b. Brachial
    c. Radial
    d. Femoral

23. Which statement about blood pressure measurement is **FALSE**?
    a. The cuff can be applied over clothing.
    b. Do not use the arm in which an IV is running.
    c. The diastolic reading is the point at which the sound disappears.
    d. Let the resident rest about 15 minutes before taking the blood pressure.

24. Which is the systolic blood pressure reading?
    a. The point where the first sound is heard.
    b. The point where the last sound is heard.
    c. The point at which the pulse is no longer felt.
    d. The point 30 mm Hg above where the pulse was felt.

25. A blood pressure consistently above normal is called
    a. heart failure.
    b. pulse deficit.
    c. hypotension.
    d. hypertension.

Chapter 11 — *Exercise, activity, and restorative care*

WORDS TO REMEMBER

abduction Moving a body part away from the body

activities of daily living (ADL) Self-care activities a person performs daily to remain independent and to function in society

adduction Moving a body part toward the body

dorsiflexion Bending backward

extension Straightening a body part

external rotation Turning the joint outward

flexion Bending a body part

footdrop Plantar flexion

hyperextension Excessive straightening of a body part

internal rotation Turning the joint inward

plantar flexion The foot is bent; footdrop

pronation Turning downward

prosthesis An artificial replacement for a missing body part

rehabilitation The process of restoring the disabled person to the highest level of physical, psychological, social, and economic functioning possible

rotation Turning the joint

supination Turning upward

PREVENTING THE COMPLICATIONS OF BED REST

Bed rest has many useful purposes. But lack of exercise and activity can cause serious complications. Pressure sores, constipation, fecal impaction, blood clots, urinary tract infections, and pneumonia (infection of the lung) can occur. Contracture and muscle atrophy (wasting) are common problems.

A contracture is the abnormal shortening of a muscle. This is a permanent deformity that must be prevented. Positioning in good body alignment is essential. Performing range-of-motion exercises is another preventive measure.

Several supportive devices can help keep the resident in good body alignment. Bed boards may be placed under the mattress to prevent it from sagging. A footboard can be placed at the foot of the mattress to prevent footdrop (plantar flexion). The footboard can also serve as a bed cradle. This keeps top linens off the person's feet.

Trochanter rolls (Fig. 8) prevent hips and legs from turning outward (external rotation). Bath blankets may also be used. Some facilities use pillows and sandbags to align the hips and legs. Thumb and finger contractures can be prevented if the person is given a handroll to grasp.

A trapeze is a bar suspended from an overbed frame. The person reaches up and grasps the trapeze with both hands to lift the trunk off the bed. Muscle strengthening exercises may be done with the trapeze.

Movement of a joint to the extent possible without causing pain is the range of motion (ROM) of that joint. ROM exercises involve exercising joints through their full range of motion. These may be active (performed by the person) exercises. Passive exercises require another person to move the joints through their range of motion. In active-assistive exercises, the person performs the exercises with some assistance. In nursing facilities, ROM exercises are part of morning care and done more frequently, if needed. (TNA 460–465; LTCA 386–393)

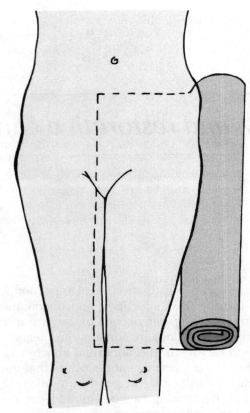

Fig. 8 A trochanter roll. (From Sorrentino SA: *Mosby's Textbook for Nursing Assistants,* ed 4, St Louis, 1996, Mosby-Year Book.)

Take note!

- Exercise only the joints that the nurse tells you to exercise.
- Expose only the body part being exercised.
- Use good body mechanics.
- Support the extremity being exercised. Move the joint slowly, smoothly, and gently. Repeat each exercise five to six times. Do not force a joint beyond its present ROM or to the point of pain.
- Perform ROM beginning with the person's neck. Then proceed downward to the shoulders, arms, hips, and legs.

Skills list

Performing Range-of-Motion Exercises (The Lower Leg), page 135

Questions for review (Answers to these questions are on page 100)

Circle the best answer.

1. Which statement about bed rest is **FALSE**?
   a. Contractures and muscle atrophy can occur.
   b. Bed rest helps reduce pain and promotes healing.
   c. Persons on bed rest are never allowed to take part in activities of daily living.
   d. Complications of bed rest include pressure sores, constipation, fecal impaction, blood clots, urinary infections, and pneumonia.

2. Which statement about contractures is **FALSE**?
   a. Contractures are permanent deformities.
   b. Contractures are an abnormal shortening of muscles.
   c. Range-of-motion exercises help prevent contractures.
   d. A contracture is a decrease in size or the wasting away of a muscle.

3. Bed boards are used to
   a. prevent plantar flexion.
   b. keep top linens off the feet.
   c. prevent the mattress from sagging.
   d. prevent the legs from rolling outward.

4. Which is used to prevent plantar flexion (foot-drop)?
   a. Handrolls
   b. Footboards
   c. Bed boards
   d. Trochanter rolls

5. The resident's hips and legs turn outward. This is
   a. abduction.
   b. adduction.
   c. internal rotation.
   d. external rotation.

6. Which is used to prevent the resident's hips from turning outward?
   a. Trapeze
   b. Footboard
   c. Bed cradle
   d. Trochanter roll

7. Footdrop and pressure ulcers of the toes and feet can both be prevented by using a
   a. trapeze.
   b. bed board.
   c. bed cradle.
   d. trochanter roll.

8. A trapeze is used for all of the following **EXCEPT**
   a. lifting the trunk off the bed.
   b. moving up and turning in bed.
   c. preventing external rotation of the hip.
   d. pulling exercises to strengthen arm muscles.

9. Passive range-of-motion exercises are performed
   a. by the resident.
   b. only by the nurse.
   c. for the resident by another person.
   d. by the resident with assistance from another person.

10. Moving a body part toward the body is called
    a. extension.
    b. adduction.
    c. abduction.
    d. supination.

11. Bending a body part is called
    a. flexion.
    b. extension.
    c. dorsiflexion.
    d. hyperextension.
12. When you move a joint during range-of-motion exercises and the person complains of pain, what should you do?
    a. Continue performing range-of-motion exercises.
    b. Stop the movement at the point the pain occurs.
    c. Give the resident pain medication before you continue.
    d. Push the resident to continue the exercises to restore movement.
13. When performing range-of-motion exercises, how often should each exercise be repeated?
    a. Once or twice
    b. Five or six times
    c. Eight or ten times
    d. Until the resident complains of being tired
14. When exercising the hip, you will move the leg away from the body. This movement is called
    a. flexion.
    b. extension.
    c. abduction.
    d. adduction.
15. When exercising the elbow, you will bend the arm so that the shoulder on the same side is touched. This movement is called
    a. flexion.
    b. extension.
    c. dorsiflexion.
    d. hyperextension.

PRESSURE SORES

Pressure sores usually occur over bony prominences. Prominence means to stick out. The shoulder blades, elbows, hip bones, sacrum, knees, ankle bones, heels, and toes are bony prominences. The first sign is pale or white skin or a reddened area. The person may complain of pain, burning, or tingling in the area. Pressure, shear, and friction are common causes of skin breakdown and pressure sores. Other factors include breaks in the skin, poor circulation to an area, moisture, dry skin, and irritation by urine and feces.

Pressure occurs when the skin over a bony prominence is squeezed between hard surfaces. The bone itself is one hard surface. The other is usually the mattress. The squeezing or pressure prevents blood flow to the skin and underlying tissues. Lack of blood flow means oxygen and nutrients cannot get to the cells, causing the involved skin and tissues to die.

Friction scrapes the skin, resulting in an open area that is a portal of entry for microorganisms. The open area needs to heal. For healing to occur, a good blood supply to the area is necessary and infection must be prevented. A poor blood supply or an infection can lead to a pressure sore.

Shearing is when the skin sticks to a surface (usually the bed or chair) and deeper tissues move downward. This occurs when a person is sitting in a chair or in Fowler's position. Shearing occurs when the person slides down in the bed or chair. The blood vessels and tissues are damaged and the blood flow to the area is reduced.

Those persons at risk for pressure sores include:
• Elderly persons
• Obese persons
• Very thin persons
• Malnourished persons
• Persons with nervous system disorders
• Persons with mobility problems
• Persons with circulatory problems

In obese people, pressure sores can develop in areas where skin is in contact with skin, resulting in friction. Pressure sores can develop between abdominal folds, the legs, the buttocks, and underneath the breasts.

Pressure ulcers develop in four stages, becoming larger with each stage.

Stage 1: Reddened skin returns to normal when pressure is relieved.

Stage 2: The skin stays reddened. Some swelling or a blister may be present.

Stage 3: The sore extends through the skin layers into underlying tissue.

Stage 4: Muscle is destroyed. The sore extends to the bone.

Pressure sores are much easier to prevent than to heal. Good nursing care, cleanliness, frequent position changes, and good skin care are essential.

The doctor may order several treatments or equipment for persons at risk for or with pressure sores. These include:

Sheepskin (lamb's wool)—Placed on the bottom sheet, it protects the skin from irritating bed linens by reducing friction between the bottom sheet and the skin. Air circulates to help keep the skin dry.

Bed cradle (Anderson frame)—A metal frame placed on the bed and over the person, it prevents pressure on the legs and feet by keeping the top linens off.

Heel and elbow protectors—Made of foam rubber or sheepskin, these fit the shape of the heel or elbow and are secured in place with straps. They prevent friction between the bed and the heel or elbow.

Flotation pads—Made of a gel-like substance with a heavy plastic outer case, these are used in chairs and wheelchairs. The pad is placed in a pillowcase so the plastic does not touch the skin.

Egg crate mattress—Peaks in this disposable foam mattress, which looks like an egg carton, distribute the person's weight more evenly. Placed on top of the regular mattress, the egg crate mattress is put in a special cover to protect against moisture and soiling. Only a bottom sheet is used to cover it.

Alternating pressure mattress—Operating electrically, it has vertical tubelike sections. Every other section is inflated with air. The other sections are deflated. Every 3 to 5 minutes the sections deflate or inflate automatically. Constant pressure on any area is avoided. Only a bottom sheet is used with it.

There are many special beds used to prevent and treat pressure sores. Some beds have air flowing through the mattress. The body weight is distributed evenly, causing the person to "float" on the bed. Another type of bed allows the person to be repositioned without moving. Depending on the bed, the person can be turned prone, supine, or tilted various degrees. Body alignment is not changed, but the pressure points change as the position changes. Some beds constantly rotate from side to side.

Trochanter rolls and footboards are also used to prevent and treat pressure sores. (TNA 314–317; LTCA 276–280)

Take note!

- Reposition the person every 2 hours. Use pillows and blankets for support, to prevent skin from being in contact with skin, and to reduce moisture and friction.
- Keep the skin clean and dry. Give perineal care as needed.
- Check with the nurse before using soap on a person at risk for pressure sores. Soap can dry and irritate the skin.
- Keep the linens clean, dry, and free of wrinkles and crumbs.
- Apply a moisturizer to dry areas such as the hands, elbows, legs, ankles, and heels.
- Give a back massage when repositioning the person.
- Do not irritate the skin. Avoid scrubbing or vigorous rubbing when bathing or drying the person.
- Massage pressure points. Use a circular motion. *Never rub or massage reddened areas.* This increases tissue damage.
- Apply powder to areas where skin touches skin. Apply lotion to dry areas such as the hands, elbows, legs, ankles, and heels. Avoid scrubbing or vigorous rubbing when bathing or drying the person's skin.

- Report any signs of skin breakdown or pressure sores immediately.
- Prevent shearing and friction during lifting and moving procedures.
- Prevent shearing by not raising the head of the bed more than 30 degrees or as instructed by the nurse.
- Remind persons sitting in chairs to shift their positions every 15 minutes to decrease pressure on body points.

Questions for review (Answers to these questions are on page 101)

Circle the best answer.

1. Which of the following are **NOT** used to treat pressure sores?
   a. Clinitron bed
   b. Heel and elbow protectors
   c. Water bed and flotation pad
   d. Plastic drawsheet and waterproof pad
2. Pressure sores most often occur
   a. over bony parts.
   b. in the stomach.
   c. in the soft, well-padded areas of the body.
   d. along the walls of the cheeks in the mouth.
3. The most common causes of pressure sores are
   a. moisture or dry skin.
   b. pressure and friction.
   c. poor circulation to an area.
   d. irritation by urine and feces.
4. Which of the following does **NOT** prevent pressure sores?
   a. Applying lotion to dry areas
   b. Scrubbing and rubbing the skin
   c. Repositioning the resident every 2 hours
   d. Keeping bed linens clean, dry, and free of wrinkles
5. Which statement about egg crate mattresses is **FALSE**?
   a. They are thrown away when soiled.
   b. They are placed under the regular mattress.
   c. Peaks in the mattress distribute the resident's weight more evenly.
   d. The bottom sheet covers both the regular and the egg crate mattress.

AMBULATION AND WALKING AIDS

Ambulation (the act of walking) is part of a progressive exercise plan for persons who have been on bed rest. Activity is increased slowly and in steps. First the person dangles (sits on the side of the bed). The next step is to sit in the bedside chair. Walking about in the room and then in the hallway are the next steps. Persons who are weak or unsteady may need help to walk. Use a gait (transfer or safety) belt when ambulating them. For additional support, ask the person to use the hand rails along the walls.

Despite every precaution, a person may begin to fall while ambulating. When a person is falling, there is a tendency to try and prevent the fall. However, trying to prevent the fall could cause more harm to you and the person. The best thing to do is to help the person to the floor. Easing the person down controls the direction of the fall. It lets you protect the person's head.

The doctor may order a walking aid to support the body. The type ordered depends on the person's physical condition, the amount of support needed, and the type of disability. The physical therapist or nurse teaches the person to use the walking aid. Crutches increase the risk of falling and are rarely used with the elderly. Canes support one side of the body and help with balance. There are single-tipped, three-point, and four-point canes. A cane is held on the *strong* side of the body. The cane tip is about 6 to 10 inches to the side of the foot and about 6 inches in front of the foot. The grip is level with the hip. The person using a cane walks as follows:

1. The cane is moved forward about 12 inches.
2. The weak leg is moved forward even with the cane.
3. The strong leg is brought forward and ahead of the cane and the weak leg. Walkers provide a safe and secure form of support. The standard walker is picked up and moved about 6 inches in front of the person. Wheeled walkers are used by persons who cannot pick up a standard walker.

Braces may be used to support a weak part, to prevent or correct deformities, or to prevent joint movement. Bony points under braces are protected. Otherwise, skin breakdown can occur. (TNA 466–472; LTCA 394–402)

Take note!

- Some persons are weak and unsteady. Use transfer (gait) belts when they ambulate and encourage them to use hand rails along the walls.
- Canes are held on the strong side of the body. Three-point and four-point canes provide more support but are much more difficult to move.
- Attach baskets, pouches, and trays as needed to walkers to allow items to be carried.

Skills list

Helping the Resident Stand and Walk, page 137

Questions for review (Answers to these questions are on page 101)

Circle the best answer.

1. You are ambulating a resident. You should
   a. encourage the resident to stand erect.
   b. encourage the resident to walk rapidly.
   c. encourage the resident to shuffle the feet.
   d. discourage the use of walking aids (canes, braces, or walkers).
2. A walker is used
   a. to support a weak body part.
   b. when one or both legs need to gain strength.
   c. to provide a safer and more secure support than a cane.
   d. to provide support when there is weakness on one side of the body.
3. You are ambulating a resident who begins to fall. You should
   a. try to steady the person.
   b. help the person to the floor.
   c. help the person back to bed.
   d. help the person to regain balance.
4. A resident is to use a single-tipped cane. Which is **INCORRECT**?
   a. The grip should be at hip level.
   b. Canes help with balance and support.
   c. The cane is moved first when walking.
   d. The cane is held on the weak side of the body.
5. How far ahead of the resident should a walker be moved for each step?
   a. 6 inches
   b. 18 inches
   c. 1 foot
   d. 2 feet
6. Braces are used for all of the following **EXCEPT** one. Which is **FALSE**?
   a. Support a weak body part
   b. Prevent movement of a joint
   c. Prevent or correct deformities
   d. Assist with range-of-motion exercises

REHABILITATION

Rehabilitation involves the whole person. It begins when the person first enters the health care facility. It requires patience, understanding, and sensitivity on the part of the health care workers. Emphasizing abilities is an important part of rehabilitation. The prevention of disabling complications is also very important.

A person's ability to perform self-care activities and the need for self-help devices are evaluated. The disabled person may or may not be totally dependent on others. Self-help devices may be needed for various activities. Equipment can usually be changed or made to meet a person's needs.

A person with a missing body part may be fitted with a prosthesis. The goal is for the prosthesis to be like the missing body part in function and appearance.

Self-esteem and relationships are often affected by a disability. Changes in appearance and function may cause the person to feel unwhole, unattractive, unclean, or undesirable to others. During the early stages of rehabilitation, the person may refuse to acknowledge the disability. The person may be depressed, angry, and hostile. Successful rehabilitation depends on the person's attitude, acceptance of limitations, and motivation. The person must focus on remaining abilities. Discouragement and frustration are common. Progress may be slow or efforts unsuccessful. The person needs help accepting the disability and the resulting limitations. Support, reassurance, encouragement, and sensitivity from the health team are necessary.

You need to observe the techniques taught to the disabled person. This will let you guide the individual more effectively during care. The more that the person can do alone, the better that person's quality of life. (TNA 569–579; LTCA 470–478)

Take note!

- Report immediately any signs or symptoms of complications. These include pressure sores, contractures, and bowel and bladder problems. Always keep the individual in good body alignment.
- Encourage the person to perform as many activities of daily living as possible and to the extent possible. Give praise when even a little progress is made.
- Make sure you can apply self-care devices or operate special equipment used by the individual. Practice for yourself the task that the individual must perform.
- Concentrate on the person's abilities, not disabilities. Do not pity or give the person sympathy. Show an attitude of hopefulness.

Questions for review (Answers to these questions are on page 101)

Circle the best answer.

1. Rehabilitation is concerned with
   a. the whole person.
   b. physical disabilities.
   c. physical capabilities.
   d. psychological and social functioning.

2. Rehabilitation emphasizes
   a. returning to normal function.
   b. the abilities of the individual.
   c. the limitations of the individual.
   d. giving complete care to the individual.

3. Rehabilitation begins when
   a. the family gives consent.
   b. the doctor gives the order.
   c. it is included in the nursing care plan.
   d. the resident enters the health care facility.

4. During rehabilitation, all of the following need to be prevented **EXCEPT**
   a. anger.
   b. contractures.
   c. pressure sores.
   d. bowel and bladder problems.

5. A prosthesis is a/an
   a. self-help device.
   b. method of rehabilitation.
   c. artificial replacement for a missing body part.
   d. solid medication that melts at body temperature.

6. The most important person on the rehabilitation team is the
   a. doctor.
   b. resident.
   c. physical therapist.
   d. occupational therapist.

7. The individual is being rehabilitated. How can you help the person overcome feelings of depression, anger, and hostility?
   a. Say that soon everything will be okay.
   b. Leave the person alone until the feelings pass.
   c. Explain how these feelings slow down progress.
   d. Give support, reassurance, and encouragement.

Chapter 12 *Special procedures and treatments*

WORDS TO REMEMBER

constrict To narrow

cyanosis Bluish discoloration of the skin

dilate To expand or open wider

embolus A blood clot that travels through the vascular system until it lodges in a distant vessel

face mask A device used to administer oxygen; it covers the nose and mouth

nasal cannula A two-pronged device used to administer oxygen; the prongs are inserted into the nostrils

saliva A thin, clear liquid produced by the salivary glands in the mouth; often called "spit"

sputum Mucus secreted by the lungs, bronchi, and trachea during respiratory illnesses or disorders

thrombus A blood clot

HEAT AND COLD APPLICATIONS

Heat and cold applications are ordered by the physician. They promote healing and comfort and reduce tissue swelling. Serious injury can occur if proper safety precautions are not taken. Some facilities do not allow nursing assistants to apply heat and cold. If you are permitted to do this, the nurse must direct the care and closely supervise the effects of the procedure.

When heat is applied to the skin, blood vessels in the area dilate (expand). More blood flows through the vessel, making more oxygen and nutrients available to the tissues for healing. The skin feels warm and appears reddened. These effects are from increased blood flow. The two main complications of heat are burns and decreased blood flow if the heat is applied for a long time. Pain, excessive redness, and blisters are danger signs. These are reported to the nurse immediately. Also observe for pale skin. When heat is applied for a long time, blood vessels tend to constrict or narrow. This decrease in the blood supply causes tissue damage and gives the skin a pale color.

Certain persons are at great risk for complications. Those at risk include:

- Elderly persons
- Persons who have difficulty sensing (feeling) heat or pain
- Persons with circulatory disorders
- Persons with central nervous system damage
- Unconscious persons
- Confused persons
- Persons receiving strong pain medication
- Persons with metal implants (pacemakers, hip and knee replacements)

Moist or dry applications are ordered. A moist heat application means that water is in contact with the skin. Since water conducts heat, the effects from moist heat are greater and occur faster than from dry heat applications. Water is not in contact with the skin with dry heat applications.

The advantages of dry heat are:

- The application stays at the desired temperature longer
- Heat is not lost through evaporation like with moist applications
- The risk of burns is less

Because water is not used, higher temperatures are needed with dry heat to achieve the desired effect. Burns are still a risk.

Hot compresses and packs are moist heat applications. A compress is applied to a small area.

Packs are applied to large areas. The compress or pack is placed in a basin of hot water. After it is wrung out, it is applied to the body part. The application is left in place for 20 minutes and then removed.

A hot soak involves putting the body part into water. The soak lasts for 15 to 20 minutes. The water temperature is checked every 5 minutes and changed as necessary. The body part is wrapped in a towel while changing the water.

The sitz bath (hip bath) involves immersing the pelvic area in warm or hot water for 20 minutes. Since the sitz bath increases blood flow to the pelvic area, the person may become weak or feel faint. The relaxing effect of the treatment may cause drowsiness. Carefully observe the person for signs of weakness, faintness, or fatigue. Hot water bottles and heat lamps are dry heat applications. An aquathermia pad uses water heated in a small unit that is pumped through channels in the pad. The temperature is set at 105° F (40.5° C) with a key provided by the manufacturer. (TNA 511–521; LTCA 430–439)

When cold is applied to the skin, blood vessels constrict or narrow. Less oxygen and nutrients are carried to the tissues. Cold is applied immediately after an injury to reduce swelling. It has a numbing effect that can relieve pain. The skin appears pale and feels cold in the area of the cold because of decreased blood flow.

Complications can occur from local cold applications. They include pain, burns and blisters, and cyanosis. When cold is applied for a long time, blood vessels tend to dilate. Blood flow increases. Those people at risk for complications from local cold applications are the elderly and persons with mental or sensory impairments.

Cold applications can be applied in a dry or moist form. Moist cold applications penetrate deeper than dry ones. Therefore temperatures of moist applications are not as cold as dry applications.

An ice bag and ice collar are dry cold applications. The bag or collar is filled with crushed ice and placed in a flannel cover. Ice bags and ice collars are left in place no longer than 30 minutes.

Disposable cold packs are dry cold applications. They are used once and discarded. A cold pack is left in place no longer than 30 minutes.

A cold compress is a moist cold application. Moist cold compresses are left in place no longer than 20 minutes.

The cool sponge bath (tepid sponge bath) is used to reduce body temperature when there is a high fever. A doctor's order is required in many facilities. The bath lasts for 25 to 30 minutes to allow time for the body to adjust. Vital signs are taken before, during, and after the procedure. They are taken every 15 minutes during the procedure. Ice bags or moist cold compresses may be used to help lower body temperature. They are applied to the forehead, axillae (underarms), and groin. (TNA 522–527; LTCA 440–445)

Take note!

- Measure the temperature of water used in moist heat applications. Follow facility policies for temperature ranges for heat applications. The following ranges are guidelines:
  Warm—93° to 98° F (33.8° to 37° C)
  Hot—98° to 105° F (37° to 40.5° C)
  Very hot—105° to 115° F (40.5° to 46.1° C)
- Cover dry heat applications with flannel protective covers before applying them to the skin.
- Observe the person's skin closely for signs of complications. Report to the nurse any complaints of pain, burning, or numbness. Also immediately report any blisters, burns, pale skin, white or gray skin, shivering, or cyanosis.
- Do not let the person change the temperature of the application. Know how long the application is to be left in place.
- Follow the rules of electrical safety when using electrical appliances to apply heat.
- Provide for the person's privacy. Expose only the body part where the heat or cold is to be applied.
- Know the correct temperature for cold applications in your facility. The following ranges are guidelines:
  Cool—65° to 80° F (18.3° to 26.6° C)
  Cold—59° to 65° F (15° to 18.3° C)
  Very cold—59° F and below (15° C or below)

Questions for review (Answers to these questions are on page 102)

Circle the best answer.
1. When heat is applied to the skin, the blood vessels
   a. dilate.
   b. narrow.
   c. contract.
   d. constrict.
2. Warm water is in contact with the skin. This is called a
   a. complication.
   b. dry heat application.
   c. local heat application.
   d. moist heat application.
3. Heat applications do all of the following **EXCEPT**
   a. relieve pain.
   b. relax muscles.
   c. promote healing.
   d. decrease blood supply.

4. The greatest danger of a heat application is
   a. loss of consciousness.
   b. the possibility of burns.
   c. an increased blood flow.
   d. damage to the central nervous system.

5. Which of these statements about moist heat applications is **FALSE**?
   a. Water is in contact with the skin.
   b. The effects are less than with a dry heat application.
   c. Heat penetrates more deeply than with a dry heat application.
   d. The temperature of the application is lower than that of a dry heat application.

6. A resident has a heat application. You observe that the skin under the application appears pale. This means
   a. the application is working.
   b. the application is not warm enough.
   c. swelling in the area is being reduced.
   d. the application has been in place too long.

7. Hot compresses are generally left in place
   a. for 5 to 10 minutes.
   b. for 20 minutes.
   c. for 2 hours.
   d. continuously.

8. Which of the following statements about sitz baths is **FALSE**?
   a. Sitz baths last 25 to 30 minutes.
   b. The pelvic area is in warm or hot water for 20 minutes.
   c. The resident may become weak or faint during the bath.
   d. Sitz baths can be used to clean the perineum, relieve pain, increase circulation, or stimulate voiding.

9. Compresses are applied to
   a. the entire body.
   b. a large body area.
   c. bruised areas only.
   d. a small area of the body.

10. Which of the following statements about heat lamps is **FALSE**?
    a. Remove the lamp after 20 to 30 minutes.
    b. Cover the lamp with bed linens for privacy.
    c. Measure the distance from the lamp to the resident.
    d. Discontinue the treatment if complications such as pain, burning, or decreased sensation occur.

11. A hot soak has been ordered. During the procedure, it is necessary to change the water because of cooling. What should you do?
    a. Wrap the part in a towel while the water is being changed.
    b. Leave the part in the cool water while you prepare another container.

c. Apply a hot compress or aquathermia pad while the water is being changed.
d. Check how much time is left and then decide if the water should be changed.

12. To protect the skin when applying a hot water bottle, the bottle is
    a. wrapped in a towel.
    b. covered with plastic.
    c. placed in a flannel cover.
    d. covered with a waterproof bed protector.

13. A hot water bottle has been applied. The cover has become moist from perspiration after 15 minutes. Which of the following is **INCORRECT**?
    a. The hot water bottle is now a moist heat application.
    b. The wet cover must be removed and a dry one applied.
    c. The resident has an increased risk for burns while the cover is moist.
    d. Moisture on the cover has no effect on the resident or the application.

14. Which of the following statements about aquathermia pads is **FALSE**?
    a. The aquathermia pad is a dry heat application.
    b. Electrical safety precautions must be practiced.
    c. Pins are used to secure the aquathermia pad in place.
    d. The temperature of the aquathermia pad is usually set at 105° F.

15. Which statement about cold applications is **INCORRECT**?
    a. Blood vessels constrict when cold is applied to the skin.
    b. Cold applications are useful immediately following an injury.
    c. Cold applications cause more oxygen and nutrients to be carried to the tissues.
    d. Cold applications reduce pain, prevent swelling, decrease circulation, and cool the body.

16. You are preparing an ice bag. You should do all of the following **EXCEPT**
    a. use ice cubes to fill the bag.
    b. fill the bag one-half to two-thirds full.
    c. place the bag in a flannel cover.
    d. remove excess air by pressing, squeezing, or twisting the bag.

17. Which is **NOT** a complication of local cold applications?
    a. Pain
    b. Cyanosis
    c. Infection
    d. Burns and blisters

18. Which of the following is a dry cold application?
    a. An ice bag
    b. A cold soak

c. A cold compress
d. A cool water bath
19. The cool water bath is ordered to
   a. relieve pain.
   b. reduce swelling.
   c. increase circulation.
   d. lower body temperature.
20. Before giving a cool sponge bath, you should
   a. measure vital signs.
   b. apply ice bags to the feet.
   c. cover the resident with several bath blankets.
   d. apply warm water bottles to the axillae and groin areas.

OXYGEN THERAPY

Oxygen is a tasteless, odorless, colorless gas. It is treated as a drug. The doctor orders the amount of oxygen to be given and the device to be used to administer the oxygen. The order states if the oxygen is to be given continuously or intermittently (periodically). Continuous oxygen therapy means that the oxygen is never stopped or interrupted for any reason. Intermittent oxygen therapy is for symptom relief. Supplemental oxygen is often ordered for acutely ill persons, those with respiratory disorders, and those with heart disease. You are never responsible for administering oxygen. However, you must give safe and effective care to persons receiving oxygen.

Oxygen is supplied through a wall outlet or by an oxygen tank. Devices used to administer oxygen include a nasal cannula or a face mask. The nasal cannula is used the most often and is the most convenient. Two prongs project from the tubing. The prongs are inserted into the nostrils. The elastic headband or tubing is brought behind the ears to keep the cannula in place. It allows the person to talk and eat while oxygen is being administered. Nasal irritation occurs if the prongs are too tight. Pressure on the ears can also occur.

Face masks cover the nose and mouth. The mask is removed for eating and drinking. Many persons experience fright and feelings of suffocation with face masks. Talking can be difficult. The person's face is kept clean and dry to help prevent irritation from the mask. (TNA 535–537; LTCA 452–455)

Take note!

- With any oxygen use, fire safety precautions must be followed exactly.
- Never shut off the flow of oxygen. Make sure there are no kinks in the tubing. Make sure the person is not lying or sitting on any part of the tubing.
- Report any sign of respiratory distress or abnormal breathing patterns to the nurse immediately.
- Give oral hygiene as directed by the nurse. Keep the resident's lips moist with petrolatum jelly.
- When using an oxygen tank, check the gauge on the tank or the fill level on the oxygen walker to see if enough oxygen is available.

Questions for review (Answers to these questions are on page 103)

Circle the best answer.
1. Which device is the simplest and most commonly used to administer oxygen?
   a. Face mask
   b. Oxygen tent
   c. Nasal cannula
   d. Nasal catheter
2. When oxygen is being used, it is most important to follow the rules related to
   a. fire safety.
   b. suctioning.
   c. medical asepsis.
   d. isolation precautions.
3. A resident is receiving supplemental oxygen. Which nursing action is **FALSE**?
   a. Give oral hygiene as directed by the nurse.
   b. Make sure there are no kinks in the tubing.
   c. Remove the administration device for meals.
   d. Follow the safety measures related to fire and the use of oxygen.
4. A resident is receiving supplemental oxygen. You may
   a. adjust the flow rate of the oxygen.
   b. give oral hygiene as directed by the nurse.
   c. turn off the oxygen until care is completed.
   d. change the face mask to a nasal cannula if the resident prefers.
5. Which statement about oxygen is **INCORRECT**?
   a. Oxygen is a drug.
   b. Oxygen is tasteless.
   c. Oxygen has a bluish color.
   d. There is no odor from oxygen.

COUGHING, DEEP BREATHING EXERCISES, AND COLLECTING SPUTUM SPECIMENS

Sputum is the mucus expelled or expectorated from the respiratory tract. In respiratory diseases, a sputum specimen is studied for blood, microorganisms, and abnormal cells. The person must cough deeply and raise sputum from the trachea and bronchi.

Coughing and deep breathing can be very painful and difficult. Some persons need to be encouraged to cough and take deep breaths while on bed rest, after surgery, or while a respiratory disorder exists. The frequency of coughing and deep breathing exercises varies. The nurse will tell you how often these exercises need to be done. (TNA 538–539; LTCA 455–458)

Take note!

- Allow privacy during these procedures. The sight and sound of collecting sputum can be unpleasant.
- Collect sputum specimens in the early morning, if possible. Let the person rinse his or her mouth with water before collecting the specimen. Do not use mouthwash because it can destroy some microorganisms that may be present.
- Place the person in a comfortable position (semi-Fowler's is preferred). Tell the person to place his or her hands over the rib cage. This gives support while coughing and deep breathing. Encourage the person to breathe in as deeply as possible through the nose. Instruct the person to hold the breath for 3 to 5 seconds and then exhale slowly through pursed lips.
- Tell the person to take a deep breath before coughing. Then tell the person to take 2 or 3 deep breaths.
- Have the person expectorate directly into the container. Sputum should not touch the outside of the container.

Questions for review (Answers to these questions are on page 103)

Circle the best answer.

1. A sputum specimen consists of secretions from
   a. the stomach.
   b. a surgical wound.
   c. the salivary glands.
   d. the lungs, trachea, and bronchi.
2. You are collecting a sputum specimen. The resident should be allowed to do all of the following **EXCEPT**
   a. void.
   b. cough five to six times.
   c. perform oral hygiene.
   d. rinse the mouth with plain water.
3. When collecting a sputum specimen, the resident should expectorate into
   a. tissues.
   b. a paper cup.
   c. an emesis basin.
   d. the specimen container.
4. The preferred position for coughing and deep breathing exercises is
   a. prone.
   b. supine.
   c. lateral.
   d. semi-Fowler's.

5. Coughing and deep breathing exercises help prevent
   a. pain.
   b. cyanosis.
   c. bleeding.
   d. respiratory complications.

BINDERS, SUPPORT BANDAGES, AND STOCKINGS

Bandages are applied to an extremity. Binders are applied to the abdomen, chest, or perineal areas. Bandages and binders are used to:

- Promote comfort
- Promote circulation
- Provide support and pressure
- Promote healing
- Prevent injury
- Hold dressings in place

They must be applied properly. Incorrect application can cause severe discomfort, skin irritation, and circulatory and respiratory complications.

There are several types of binders. Straight abdominal binders support the abdomen. T-binders secure dressings in place after rectal or perineal surgery.

Support bandages are called elastic bandages. They promote circulation or reduce swelling in extremities. Elastic stockings are ordered for persons at risk for developing thrombi (blood clots). A blood clot in a vein can break off and become an embolus (moving clot). Venous blood clots usually lodge in the lungs, resulting in severe respiratory problems and/or death.

Elastic stockings are often called TED hose or AE (antiembolic stockings). They help prevent the development of thrombi by exerting pressure on the veins. This promotes venous blood flow to the heart. The nurse measures the person to determine proper size. The stockings are applied before the person gets out of bed and are removed at least twice a day. (TNA 560–563; LTCA 459–462)

Take note!

- Apply binders and bandages so that firm, even pressure is exerted over the area. They should fit snugly, yet not interfere with breathing or circulation. The body must be in good alignment.
- Reapply a binder or bandage if it is loose, wrinkled, moist, soiled, or out of position.
- Leave toes or fingers exposed, if possible, when applying an elastic bandage. Check the color and temperature of the extremity every hour.

Skills list

Applying Knee-Length Elastic Stockings, page 140

Questions for review (Answers to these questions are on page 103)

Circle the best answer.

1. Binders are applied to
   a. prevent wound infections.
   b. prevent blood clots in the legs.
   c. decrease circulation and swelling.
   d. provide support or hold dressings in place.
2. Elastic stockings are worn to
   a. increase swelling.
   b. increase venous blood flow.
   c. decrease venous blood flow.
   d. encourage blood clot formation.
3. A blood clot that travels through the vascular system until it lodges in a distant vessel is called a/an
   a. embolus.
   b. thrombi.
   c. thrombus.
   d. antiembolus.
4. A binder is loose and wrinkled. You should
   a. change the binder.
   b. reapply the binder.
   c. remove the binder and leave it off.
   d. secure the binder with additional pins.
5. Elastic stockings are
   a. removed once a day.
   b. available in one size only.
   c. applied after the person has been up for 20 minutes.
   d. available in many sizes so the nurse measures the person to determine the correct size.

CLEARING AN OBSTRUCTED AIRWAY (HEIMLICH MANEUVER)

Obstruction of the airway (choking) can lead to cardiac arrest. This is the sudden stoppage of breathing and heart action. Air cannot pass through the air passages to the lungs. The entire body is deprived of oxygen. Airway obstruction often occurs while eating. Meat is the most common cause of choking. Other causes include improperly fitting dentures, hard candy, apples, or pieces of hot dogs. In the unconscious person, aspiration of vomitus and the tongue falling back into the airway can cause obstruction. Weakness, chronic illnesses, and poor swallowing reflexes can also result in choking in the elderly.

When airway obstruction occurs, the victim will clutch at the throat. The victim cannot breathe, speak, or cough, appears pale and cyanotic, and will be very apprehensive if conscious. The obstruction must be removed immediately.

The Heimlich maneuver, which involves abdominal thrusts, is recommended for relieving an obstructed airway. The maneuver can be done with the victim standing, sitting, or lying down. However, it is not effective in the obese person. Chest thrusts are used instead. The finger sweep is an additional maneuver used when the victim is unconscious. You need to activate the Emergency Medical System (EMS) when a victim has an obstructed airway. (TNA 696–701; LTCA 543–545)

Take note!

- The Heimlich maneuver—conscious adult
  a. Ask if victim is choking.
  b. Determine if the victim can cough or speak.
  c. The victim is standing or sitting.
     (1) Stand behind the victim.
     (2) Wrap your arms around the victim's waist.
     (3) Make a fist with one hand. Place the thumb side of the fist against the abdomen. The fist is in the middle above the navel and below the sternum.
     (4) Grasp your fist with your other hand.
     (5) Press your fist and hand into the victim's abdomen with a quick, upward thrust.
     (6) Repeat until the object is expelled or the victim loses consciousness.
- Chest thrusts
  a. The victim is sitting or standing.
  b. Stand behind the victim.
  c. Place your arms under the victim's arms. Wrap your arms around the victim's chest.
  d. Make a fist. Place the thumb side of the fist on the middle of the sternum.
  e. Grasp the fist with your other hand.
  f. Give backward chest thrusts until the object is expelled or the victim becomes unconscious.

Skills list

Clearing the Obstructed Airway (Heimlich Maneuver)—The Conscious Adult, page 141

Questions for review (Answers to these questions are on page 104)

Circle the best answer.

1. The most common food to cause an airway obstruction is
   a. meat.
   b. liquids.
   c. small peas.
   d. applesauce.
2. A resident who is choking will
   a. appear flushed.
   b. say he is choking.
   c. clutch at the throat.
   d. take short, quick breaths.

3. The Heimlich maneuver is not effective if the resident is
   a. obese.
   b. sitting.
   c. standing.
   d. lying down.
4. When performing the Heimlich maneuver on a victim who is standing, you should do all of the following **EXCEPT**
   a. stand behind the victim.
   b. wrap your hands around the victim's waist.
   c. place your fist in the middle of the abdomen above the navel and below the sternum.
   d. press your fist and hand into the victim's abdomen and give quick, downward thrusts.
5. Which of the following is **NOT** a cause of choking in the elderly?
   a. Weakness
   b. Chronic illnesses
   c. Properly fitting dentures
   d. Poor swallowing reflexes

CHAPTER 1
The nursing assistant
Nursing Assistants in Long-Term Care
(pp. 9–10)

1. **C**   Always ask the nurse if you have questions about a procedure or what is expected of you. The nurse is your supervisor. Do not attempt a task for which you have not been adequately prepared. Asking the resident how to perform a procedure is inappropriate. While you should never refuse or ignore a request, you need to know the limits of your role and knowledge. Nor can you perform any act that is not within the legal scope of the nursing assistant. (TNA 19; LTCA 14–15)

2. **A**   Nursing assistants are *never* allowed to give medications. That requires knowledge about drugs and their actions. Nursing assistants may not supervise other nursing assistants. Nursing assistants do perform personal hygiene tasks for residents. Nurses make decisions about resident care. The nurse is your supervisor. However, do not attempt a task for which you have not been adequately prepared. You need to know the limits of your role and knowledge. Remember, you cannot perform any act that is not within the legal scope of the nursing assistant.

3. **A**   The physician informs the resident and family about the resident's diagnosis and treatment. Nurses may further explain this information to the resident or the family. Other staff members and nursing assistants need to recognize the limits of their roles and knowledge. (TNA 18–24; LTCA 18–19)

4. **B**   You must always respect the resident's beliefs or values. Nursing assistants must be careful, alert, and exact in following orders and instructions. Reporting care, observations, and measurements accurately allows you to provide thorough care with knowledge and skill. Knowing your own feelings, strengths, and weaknesses helps you understand others. (TNA 18–24; LTCA 18–19)

5. **A**   Planning care requires that you consider many factors. Review the procedures to be performed and gather the necessary supplies beforehand. This will save you time and enable you to provide safe, thorough care. Listing care or procedures to be performed enables you to set priorities. Setting priorities is essential. Give attention to the most important tasks first. Being flexible lets you work around such things as meals, activities, and room availability. You may need to plan care when other staff members can help. (TNA 38–40; LTCA 23–24)

Legal Considerations
(p. 11)

1. **A**   Assault is intentionally attempting or threatening to touch a person's body without the person's consent. Battery is the actual unauthorized touching of another person's body without the person's consent. Defamation is injuring the name and reputation of another person by making false statements to a third person. False imprisonment is the unlawful restraint or restriction of a person's freedom of movement. (TNA 26–28; LTCA 21–23)

2. **C**   Since the resident's complaint of chest pain and difficulty breathing was reported to the nurse, the nursing assistant was not negligent. Negligence occurs when the person fails to act in a reasonable and careful manner and as a result causes harm to the person or the person's property. Dropping the resident's dentures and breaking them is negligence. Not checking the temperature of a warm water bottle and burning a

resident is negligence. The nursing assistant is negligent when side rails, which were ordered for a confused resident, are left down and the resident falls, breaking a hip.

3. **A** Threatening to touch a person's body without the person's consent is assault. Telling the resident that she will have a bath whether she likes it or not causes the resident to fear bodily harm. Giving the resident the bath without her consent would be battery. Battery is the actual touching of a person's body without the person's consent. Defamation has not occurred because the name and reputation of the resident has not been injured by false statements to a third person. False imprisonment has not occurred since the resident's freedom of movement has not been restrained or restricted. (TNA 26–28; LTCA 21–23)

4. **C** You are legally responsible for your own actions. While the nurse will be held liable as your supervisor, in no way are you relieved of personal liability. You cannot perform any act that is not within the legal scope of the nursing assistant. You need to know the limits of your role and knowledge. While you function under the direction and supervision of the nurse, there are times that you have a right and a duty to refuse to follow the nurse's directions. In this situation the nurse's directions are unethical, illegal, and against the policies of the facility. (TNA 26–28; LTCA 21–23)

5. **B** When negligence occurs, harm is caused to a person or a person's property. Negligence is an unintentional tort. The negligent person failed to act in a reasonable and careful manner. As a nursing assistant, you are legally responsible (liable) for your own actions. (TNA 26–28; LTCA 21–23)

Resident Rights
(p. 12)

1. **B** Opening resident's mail, searching personal items without permission, and requiring the resident to remain in view while visiting are invasions of privacy. (TNA 140–143; LTCA 8–10)

2. **B** False imprisonment is the unlawful restraint or restriction of a person's freedom of movement. Using restraints to prevent a person from leaving the facility is an example of false imprisonment. OBRA states that residents have the right to be free from verbal, sexual, physical, or mental abuse. Activities are important to a resident's quality of life. OBRA requires that nursing facilities provide activity programs that meet the interests and physical, mental, and psychosocial needs of each resident. Residents have the right to participate in planning their own care and treatment. Personal choice is important for quality of life, dignity, and self-respect. (TNA 140–143; LTCA 8–10)

3. **C** OBRA does not require the resident to have a private room. Courteous and dignified interactions with residents are required by OBRA. Residents also have the right to visit with others in private. The environment of the facility must be clean, safe, and as home-like as possible. (TNA 140–143; LTCA 8–10)

4. **C** Residents have the right to make decisions about their own care and treatment. This means that the resident has the right to choose when to get up and go to bed, what to wear, how to spend their time, what to eat, and how their hair should be styled. The nurse should ask the resident how he or she prefers the hair to be styled. If the resident is unable to make decisions or state what he or she would prefer, the family may be asked. The nursing assistant should ask the resident what he or she would prefer. (TNA 140–143; LTCA 8–10)

5. **C** Assisting the resident to and from activity programs promotes the resident's quality of life. Residents have the right to keep and use personal possessions. Residents have the right to choose what activities they want to attend. Courteous and dignified care of the resident is promoted by a neat and clean appearance. (TNA 140–143; LTCA 8–10)

Privacy and Confidentiality
(p. 13)

1. **D** The condition and treatment of residents must be discussed only by those workers directly involved in their care. Working in a facility does not give one access to privileged information. Making sure the resident is covered when being moved in corridors protects the resident's right to privacy. Screening the person and closing the door when giving care ensures the resident's privacy. Exposing only the body part involved in a treatment or procedure treats the resident with respect and ensures the resident's privacy. (TNA 28; LTCA 8–9)

2. **D** Residents should be allowed to visit with others and to use the telephone in private. Visitors should be asked to leave the room when care must be given. Only personnel involved in the person's care should be present when care is given. Only the body part involved in a treatment or procedure should be exposed. Make sure the person is covered when being moved in corridors. (TNA 141; LTCA 8–9)

3. **D** Information about the resident's care, treatment, and condition must be kept confidential.

Only those members of the health care team involved in the resident's care have access to the chart. Health care team members record information on the forms for their department and service. Many facilities will allow residents to see their records if they request it. The nurse is responsible for handling a resident's request to see his or her medical record. Those health care workers not directly involved in the resident's care usually cannot review the person's record. (TNA 28; LTCA 8–9)

4. **B** Residents have the right to privacy. This right to privacy includes telephone conversations. Opening the resident's mail is an invasion of privacy. Residents have the right to send and receive mail without interference by others. Searching the resident's closet and drawers is an invasion of privacy. The security of the resident's personal possessions would also be questionable. Residents have the right to visit with others in private. They have the right to visit in an area where they cannot be seen or heard by others. (TNA 28; LTCA 8–9)

CHAPTER 2
Communication

Communication Among the Health Care Team
(pp. 15–16)

1. **A** A message sent, received, and interpreted by the intended person is communication. It is an exchange. Communication can be written or verbal. All of the senses are used in communication. Communication occurs through reporting as well as recording information. (TNA 45; LTCA 28)

2. **B** The main reason for the resident's record is to provide a way for the health care team to communicate information about the person. It can be used in court as evidence of the resident's problems, treatment, and care. The record is permanent and can be retrieved years later if the person's health history is needed. While many facilities let residents see their records if they request it, residents and families are not given the record. (TNA 46–47; LTCA 29–32)

3. **D** Each page must be stamped with the resident's name, room number, and other identifying information. Identifying each page reduces the possibility of errors and improper placement of records. The record has many forms organized into sections. Not all pages will be numbered. Health care team members record information on the forms for their department and service. Every page does not have to be signed by the doctor. (TNA 46–47; LTCA 29–32)

4. **D** Only those health care workers involved in the resident's care need to see the chart. Many facilities let residents and families see the records if they so request. Those health care workers not directly involved in the resident's care usually cannot read the resident's chart. The physicians and nurses involved in the person's care have access to the chart. (TNA 46–47; LTCA 29–32)

5. **B** Always use ink to record information. Pencil can be erased or smudged. Do not skip lines. Lines are drawn through the blank space of a partially completed line or to the end of the page. This prevents others from recording in a space with your signature. The date and time are included whenever an entry is made in the chart. All entries are signed with your name and title according to your facility's policy. Each entry is signed, dated, and timed. (TNA 64–66; LTCA 32–37)

6. **D** The nursing care plan is a written guide that gives direction about the care a resident should receive. The Kardex summarizes the information found in the medical record. The nurse writes the nursing care plan. Nursing measures may come from a doctor's order or from input from other health care team members. Care plans are developed for each resident to assist in meeting his or her goals. (TNA 45)

7. **C** Information the resident tells you that you cannot observe through your senses is subjective data. Information or data that you can observe is objective data. Collective data is not a term used in health care. Comprehensive data is not a term used in health care. (TNA 53; LTCA 35)

8. **B** The Kardex is a quick reference for routines. It would be appropriate to ask the nurse. The information would be included in the nurse's notes, but would not be found as quickly. The physical therapy report would have this information but would not be found as quickly. (TNA 47; LTCA 43)

9. **A** Errors in charting are not erased. They are identified by a single line drawn through the word or words with "error" written above it. Each entry is signed with your name and title as required by facility policy. Use the resident's exact words whenever possible. Use quotation marks to show that the statement is a direct quote. Only chart after a procedure or treatment has been completed. (TNA 64–66; LTCA 32–37)

10. **D** Reports are given as often as the resident's condition requires or as requested by the nurse. At the beginning of the shift, the oncoming shift is given a report from the shift that is leaving. The care given and observations made are reported at the end of the shift to assist the nurse in his or her report. (LTCA 32–37; TNA 64–66)

The Hearing Impaired Resident
(pp. 16–17)

1. **B** Loneliness and boredom are not signs of hearing loss. Persons with hearing impairment will speak too loudly, ask for things to be repeated, and answer inappropriately. (TNA 584–587; LTCA 499–500)
2. **A** Hearing aids make all sounds louder, including background noise. They do not make speech clearer, nor do they correct hearing problems. (TNA 584–587; LTCA 499–500)
3. **A** Do not shout. Speak slowly in a normal tone of voice. Face the person so he or she can read your lips and see your expression. (TNA 584–587; LTCA 499–500)
4. **B** Only the removable earpiece can be washed gently in soap and water. Do not use hot water or alcohol because it could warp or damage the earmold. Never soak the entire hearing aid because water could damage it. Hearing aids are expensive and must be handled carefully and cared for properly to prevent breaking them. (TNA 584–587; LTCA 499–500)
5. **D** Do not cover your mouth, smoke, or chew gum while talking. These actions affect mouth movements. Stating the topic of discussion, writing out important names and words, and using short sentences and simple words are appropriate actions. (TNA 584–587; LTCA 499–500)

Medical Terminology
(pp. 17–18)

1. **A** Hemiplegia is paralysis on one side of the body. Paraplegia is paralysis from the waist down. Hemaplegia is an incorrect spelling. Quadriplegia is paralysis from the neck down. (TNA 739–745; LTCA 568–572)
2. **A** The medical abbreviation for before meals is "ac." After meals is "pc." "BM" is the abbreviation for bowel movement. "NPO" means nothing by mouth. (TNA 739–745; LTCA 568–572)
3. **C** The medical abbreviation "prn" means when necessary. As desired is "ad lib." The medical abbreviation for immediately is "stat." There is no medical abbreviation that means "patient really needs." (TNA 739–745; LTCA 568–572)
4. **B** The medical abbreviation for twice a day is "bid." Every day is "qd." Three times a day is "tid." Four times a day is "qid." (TNA 739–745; LTCA 568–572)
5. **B** The medical abbreviation "qod" means every other day. The medical abbreviation for every day is "qd." Four times a day is "qid." Every four hours is "q4h." (TNA 739–745; LTCA 568–572)

CHAPTER 3
Understanding the person
Basic Needs
(pp. 19–20)

1. **D** To effectively care for the whole person we need to see the physical, psychological, social, and spiritual parts woven together. The person's body cannot be separated from the other parts. Each part relates to and depends on the others. The resident's view of himself or herself is important, but the health care worker needs to care for the total person. The resident should not be treated as a physical disease, problem, or room and bed number. (TNA 75–77; LTCA 50–52)
2. **B** Mr. Michaels is confused and frightened. This affects safety and security needs. Physiological needs are those needs necessary for survival. The need for love and belonging relate to meaningful relationships with others. Esteem needs are the resident's opinion and feelings of self-worth. (TNA 75–77; LTCA 50–52)
3. **D** Mrs. Smith does not see herself as useful or valuable. This affects her self-esteem. Physiological needs are those needs necessary for survival. Safety and security needs relate to the need to feel free from harm or danger. The need for love and belonging relate to meaningful relationships with others. Esteem needs are the resident's opinion and feelings of self-worth. (TNA 75–77; LTCA 50–52)
4. **C** Feeling isolated, alone, with few or no meaningful relationships affects the need for love and belonging. Physiological needs are those needs necessary for survival. Safety and security needs relate to the need to feel free from harm or danger. Esteem needs are the resident's opinion and feelings of self-worth. (TNA 75–77; LTCA 50–52)
5. **D** Mrs. Adams is showing a desire to be creative. This involves the need for self-actualization. Physiological needs are those needs necessary for survival. Safety and security needs relate to the need to feel free from harm or danger. The need for love and belonging relates to meaningful relationships with others. (TNA 75–77; LTCA 50–52)

Culture and Religion
(p. 20)

1. **B** Mrs. Greene's refusal reflects her religious beliefs. The nurse and the dietician can assist her in selecting a diet that will meet her religious dietary restrictions. It would not be appropriate for the nursing assistant to notify the doctor. Telling the resident that she will not receive any-

thing else to eat could be considered assault. The resident has the right to make decisions about her own care and treatment. This is important for the resident's quality of life, dignity, and self-respect. (TNA 77; LTCA 52)

2. **C** By listening to Mr. O'Malley, the nursing assistant will learn about his cultural beliefs and health care practices. Changing the subject does not give the nursing assistant the opportunity to understand the resident and give better care. By talking about his or her family, the nursing assistant is not putting the resident's needs first. The nurse will need to be notified only if the resident's health care will be affected after resident care is completed. (TNA 77; LTCA 52)

3. **D** Learning as much as you can about the resident's cultural beliefs and health care practices will enable you to provide care that meets the resident's needs. It is important because culture influences behavior during illness. In the health care facility, the resident's care plan includes measures that include the resident's cultural and religious practices. Learning about the resident's culture is important regardless of whether the resident has family or friends because culture influences health and illness practices. (TNA 77; LTCA 52)

4. **C** The nurse needs to know about Mrs. Johnson's request. She decides which clergy member to call. (TNA 77; LTCA 52)

5. **C** The nurse and resident will plan measures that will include the resident's cultural and religious practices. Both cultural and religious beliefs may influence dietary practices. The person's culture influences health beliefs and practices. Individuals may not follow every belief and practice of their culture or religion. (TNA 77; LTCA 52)

Social Functioning
(p. 21)

1. **A** Aging is a natural, normal process. The rate and degree will vary with each person. Injury may accompany the normal changes of aging. Diseases may occur as a part of aging. Illness may accompany aging as part of the normal changes that occur. (TNA 133; LTCA 96)

2. **A** Retirement usually means reduced financial income. Some individuals feel worthless and lack self-esteem without work, which results in social emptiness. Retirement may cause the person's sense of pride that resulted from work to be replaced with feelings of uselessness. (TNA 133–134; LTCA 96)

3. **C** When elderly parents move in with adult children, tension often develops because of a lack of privacy. While the father may feel more secure,

he may also feel a loss of control. There will be a reversal of parent-child roles. Some elderly persons feel a loss of dignity and self-respect. (TNA 135; LTCA 99)

4. **A** In general, men do not live as long as women. The surviving spouse may lose the will to live or attempt suicide. It is common for surviving spouses to develop serious physical health problems. The surviving spouse may develop serious mental health problems. (TNA 135; LTCA 99)

5. **C** Family and friends are not responsible for giving care to residents. Visits from family and friends can help recovery by meeting the resident's need for love and belonging. Family and friends offer the resident comfort and support. The resident's safety, security, love and belonging needs are met by family and friends. (TNA 134–135; LTCA 99)

Sexuality and the Elderly
(pp. 21–22)

1. **C** Let the resident choose what clothing he or she wants to wear. Hospital gowns are embarrassing to both men and women. Allowing the person to practice grooming routines promotes his or her sexuality. Accept the resident's sexual relationships. Allow the resident privacy when it is needed. (TNA 659; LTCA 526–532)

2. **D** Impotence is the inability of the male to have an erection. Impotence is not always permanent. Abstinence is the absence of sexual activity. Menopause is when the menstrual cycle stops. (TNA 658; LTCA 526–532)

3. **A** Menopause is when the menstrual cycle stops. Impotence is the inability of the male to have an erection. Sex consists of the physical activities involving the organs of reproduction. Sexuality is those physical, psychological, social, cultural, and spiritual factors that affect a person's feelings and attitudes about sex. (TNA 659; LTCA 526–532)

4. **C** Allow for the resident's privacy and safety if the resident is masturbating. Providing for safety involves raising the side rails and placing the signal light within reach. Tell the resident when you will return. There is no need to tell the nurse because it is a normal form of sexual expression and release. Continuing as if nothing has happened does not allow the resident privacy. It would not be appropriate to tell the resident that his or her behavior makes you uncomfortable because this is a normal form of sexual expression and release. (TNA 660; LTCA 526–532)

5. **D** We cannot make judgments about a resident's relationships. The person's selection of partners may not align with our personal moral

standards. Knocking before you enter a room is a common courtesy and shows respect for privacy. Residents need to be allowed to select their own clothing. Residents should be encouraged to practice personal grooming routines. (TNA 660; LTCA 526–532)

The Dying Person
(pp. 22–23)

1. **C**   Terminal illness is one from which a person is not expected to recover. An acute illness is one in which a person will recover. Chronic illnesses continue a long time, but do not usually cause death. Long-term illness is another name for chronic illnesses. (TNA 711–721; LTCA 556–564)
2. **D**   Hearing is the last sense lost during the dying process. Taste is affected by any increase of mucus in the mouth. Vision becomes blurred and gradually fails during the dying process. Smell may be affected by the crusting and irritation of the nostrils. (TNA 714; LTCA 556–564)
3. **B**   Family is usually allowed to spend as much time as possible with the loved one. Family members can help give care if they wish. Normal visiting hours do not apply if the person is dying. The resident's care cannot be neglected because the family is present. (TNA 715; LTCA 558)
4. **D**   Ask questions that can be answered "yes" or "no." The nursing team needs to anticipate the person's needs. Do not ignore the resident or deny the chance to communicate. Most dying persons are too weak to write messages. (TNA 714; LTCA 558)
5. **B**   The "death rattle" is a result of mucus collecting in the respiratory passages as death approaches. There are no vital signs when the resident is dead. (TNA 717; LTCA 559)
6. **D**   The extremities farthest from the vital organs (heart, brain, kidney, liver) show signs of approaching death first. This slowly spreads upward through the body. (TNA 717; LTCA 559)
7. **D**   Secretions tend to accumulate and form crusts around the mouth and nose. These secretions are not affected by food intake. Mouth care is important for comfort and needs to be given often. (TNA 714–715; LTCA 558)
8. **C**   Rigor mortis begins 2 to 4 hours after death. It is a result of chemical changes in muscle fibers. It is a gradual process that is complete within 8 hours after death. (TNA 717; LTCA 559)
9. **C**   Postmortem care begins as soon as the doctor pronounces the person dead. Postmortem care involves positioning the body in normal alignment before rigor mortis sets in. Postmortem care is done to maintain the body's ap-

pearance. If the family wants to see the body, it should appear in a comfortable and natural position. Postmortem care is completed later by the funeral director. (TNA 717; LTCA 559)
10. **D**   Persons in denial refuse to believe they are dying. People feeling anger and rage are in the stage of anger. Being sad and quiet indicates the person is in depression. Bargaining is the stage where the person bargains with God for more time. (TNA 712; LTCA 557)

CHAPTER 4
Safety
The Safe Environment
(pp. 25–26)

1. **A**   Accidents in long-term care facilities most often involve falls by residents. This is because many elderly residents cannot see or move independently. While burns are a leading cause of death in the elderly, they occur less often than falls. Accidental poisoning is another major cause of death but occurs less often than falls. Suffocation occurs less often than falls. (TNA 158; LTCA 114)
2. **B**   Residents are allowed to use heating pads only when ordered by a doctor and with supervision. A resident may fall asleep during the day or evening. Not allowing smoking in bed reduces the risk of burns. Measuring the temperature of the bath water helps to prevent burns. Removing smoking materials and supervising the smoking of adults who cannot protect themselves reduces the risk of burns. (LTCA 114; TNA 511)
3. **B**   The edges of throw rugs can easily turn up or catch one's heels. The elderly are often unable to see danger because of poor vision. Handrails on both sides of stairs and in bathrooms are a safety measure to prevent falls. Nonskid shoes and slippers help residents move about safely. A telephone and lamp at the bedside do not pose a problem unless electrical cords get in the way. (TNA 158–161; LTCA 115–116)
4. **C**   The identification bracelet is the most reliable way to identify a resident. The nurse may be new and unfamiliar with the residents. Some residents will answer to other names. Residents can move about and may not be found in their own rooms. (TNA 158; LTCA 113)
5. **D**   A resident who is alert and can be permitted to ambulate around the facility does not need the side rails raised. Residents who are confused may need to have their side rails elevated. Side rails remain elevated for residents who are comatose. Residents who are sedated

with medication need to have their side rails elevated. (TNA 159; LTCA 114–115)

6. **D** The bed should always be kept in the lowest horizontal position except when giving care. Residents should always wear nonskid shoes. A nightlight assists the resident in moving about the room safely. The signal light must always be within the resident's reach. (TNA 157–163; LTCA 113–126)

7. **B** As soon as you notice an electrical hazard, report it to the nurse. Do not attempt to change to a different cord. This must be done by properly trained personnel in the maintenance department. Stop using the equipment and report it. (TNA 174; LTCA 129–130)

8. **D** Gas leaks can quickly lead to danger. First remove the resident and yourself from the area. Then report the odor according to the facility's policy. Time is very important. Gas odors should be promptly investigated by competent repairmen.

9. **D** Report the incident to the nurse immediately. The nurse needs to know about an incident because it may or may not affect the resident's condition. Measures may need to be taken immediately. An incident report must also be completed. The treatment can be given to the right resident after informing the nurse. (TNA 174; LTCA 128–129)

10. **A** The comatose resident is completely helpless. Age is not always a factor in one's ability to protect himself. (TNA 153; LTCA 112)

Protective Devices (Restraints)
(pp. 26–27)

1. **B** Some movement is allowed when restraints are used. This insures that the restraint is not too tight. A doctor's order is required for restraints. Always protect bony areas with padding. Many residents become agitated when restrained. (TNA 160–173; LTCA 116–127)

2. **B** The nurse knows why the restraints were used. Report the time of the application. The type of restraint used needs to be reported. Any care given when the restraints were removed is reported to the nurse. (TNA 160–173; LTCA 116–127)

3. **C** The restraint is removed and the resident repositioned every 2 hours. Less time may not be possible. More than 2 hours is too long for the resident to be in one position. (TNA 160–173; LTCA 116–127)

4. **B** Difficulty breathing requires immediate attention. Restraints are secured to the movable part of the bed frame. Residents will pull at restraints. The resident's fingers and toes should be warm and pink. (TNA 160–173; LTCA 116–127)

5. **A** Restraints are used to protect the person, not for staff convenience. Using a restraint to prevent a resident from falling out of bed would be appropriate. Restraints are used to protect persons from harming themselves or others. Using restraints to prevent a resident from pulling out tubes or disconnecting equipment would be appropriate. (TNA 160–173; LTCA 116–127)

6. **B** The vest never crosses in the back. When the straps are in the back, the jacket can slide up around the resident's neck and cause strangulation. The vest is always applied over clothing. The bed frame is used to secure the tie. The resident should be comfortable and in good body alignment. (TNA 160–173; LTCA 116–127)

7. **C** The nurse needs to check the resident immediately to decide if the restraint should be removed or readjusted. You must not assume this responsibility yourself. (TNA 160–173; LTCA 116–127)

8. **D** Removing the restraint, giving skin care, and repositioning the resident every 2 hours helps promote quality of life. Leaving the restraints in place over an extended period of time limits the resident's ability to meet basic needs. The care plan should show how the use of restraints will be decreased. The resident's joints should be given range-of-motion exercises every 2 hours. (TNA 160–173; LTCA 116–127)

Fire Safety
(p. 28)

1. **A** Oxygen is essential for fires. Its use requires very special precautions for fire safety. Heat treatments place the resident at risk for burns. Intravenous medications will not cause a fire. Sleeping medications only pose a fire risk if the resident smokes while sedated. (TNA 175–176; LTCA 129–130)

2. **C** Three-pronged electrical plugs provide a ground and are safer to use. A frayed cord can be the cause of a fire. Overloaded electrical circuits are a major cause of fires. Electrical equipment that gives off shocks is a hazard. (TNA 174; LTCA 128)

3. **D** Electrical items must be removed from an area where oxygen is used as a safety precaution to prevent sparks. Wool and synthetic fabrics must be removed from an area where oxygen is used. This is a safety precaution since wool and synthetic fibers cause static electricity, which may produce sparks. The no-smoking policy is strictly enforced. All electrical switches must be turned off before unplugging. Sparks occur when electrical appliances are unplugged while turned on. (TNA 175; LTCA 129)

4. **A** Since the alarm has already sounded, the first thing you should do is locate the fire. There is no need to pull the alarm again. After the fire has been located, a fire extinguisher can be taken to the scene. A determination as to whether residents should be evacuated is based on the extent of the fire. (TNA 175–176; LTCA 129)

5. **C** Residents should not be moved unless they are in immediate danger from smoke or flames. All equipment is cleared from all regular and emergency exits. All windows and doors are closed to control ventilation. Elevators are not used if there is a fire. (TNA 175–176; LTCA 129)

6. **C** The extinguisher is aimed at the base or source of the fire. Otherwise, the fire may spread. (TNA 176; LTCA 130)

CHAPTER 5
Infection control
Medical Asepsis
(p. 32)

1. **B** Light and heat destroy microorganisms. The microbe must get nourishment from the reservoir (host). Water is necessary for the microorganism. A warm, dark environment is needed for microbes to grow. (TNA 183–184; LTCA 136)

2. **A** Pathogens are microorganisms that are harmful and capable of causing an infection. Protozoa are microscopic one-celled animals. Not all protozoa are pathogenic. Bacteria are one-celled microorganisms that multiply rapidly. Not all bacteria are pathogenic. Nonpathogens do not cause disease. (TNA 183–184; LTCA 136)

3. **D** Medical asepsis is the term used to describe these techniques. Sterilization kills all organisms. Handwashing is a technique of medical asepsis. Contamination is when an object becomes unclean.

4. **C** Contamination is when an object becomes unclean. Sterilization kills all organisms. Disinfection is the process by which pathogens are destroyed. Medical asepsis is the techniques and practices used to prevent the spread of pathogens from one person or place to another person or place. (TNA 183; LTCA 135)

5. **A** Sterilization kills all organisms. Disinfection is the process by which pathogens are destroyed. Contamination is when an object becomes unclean. Medical asepsis is the techniques and practices used to prevent the spread of pathogens from one person or place to another person or place. (TNA 183; LTCA 135)

6. **D** The sink is considered dirty. Do not let your uniform touch the sink. Stand at a reasonable distance so you can reach the faucets and the soap. (TNA 187–188; LTCA 137–139)

7. **A** Handwashing needs to last about 1 to 2 minutes. Any longer amount of time would not be realistic for routine handwashing during resident care. (TNA 187–188; LTCA 137–139)

8. **D** The faucet is usually considered dirty. Use a clean, dry paper towel to turn the water off. This prevents your hands from becoming contaminated. Then discard the towel. The sink is not cleaned at this time. (TNA 187–188; LTCA 137–139)

9. **A** Always rinse items in cold water to remove organic material. A brush can be used to clean equipment, but it is not used first. Hot water makes it very difficult to remove organic waste. It is your responsibility to clean used equipment. (TNA 189–190; LTCA 140)

10. **D** Handwashing is an example of medical asepsis. Handwashing with soap and water is the easiest and the single most effective way to prevent the spread of infection. Sterilization is the process by which all microorganisms are destroyed. Disinfection is the process by which pathogens are destroyed. Contamination is the process by which an object or area becomes unclean. (TNA 187–188; LTCA 137–139)

Communicable Disease Control
(pp. 33–34)

1. **B** Residents with contagious (communicable) diseases require isolation precautions. Allergies are not contagious. Not all infections are contagious. Not all gastrointestinal diseases are caused by contagious pathogens. (TNA 192; LTCA 142)

2. **D** Gowns and gloves are worn when direct contact with the wound or drainage is expected. Masks prevent the spread of microbes from the respiratory tract. Gowns are worn when direct contact with the wound or drainage is expected. Gloves are worn whenever contact with blood or with body fluids, body substances, or mucous membranes that contain blood or infectious material is possible. (TNA 196–199; LTCA 144–146)

3. **A** Enteric precautions prevent the spread of pathogens through fecal material. Contact precautions prevent the spread of infection by close or direct contact. Universal precautions deal with blood and body fluids. Respiratory precautions prevent the spread of pathogens through the air. (TNA 194–195; LTCA 142)

4. **B** Respiratory isolation prevents the spread of pathogens through the air. Enteric precautions

prevent the spread of pathogens through fecal material. Drainage isolation prevents the spread of pathogens in wounds or wound drainage. Contact isolation prevents the spread of infection by close or direct contact. (TNA 194–195; LTCA 142)

5. **D** Gloves are used to handle contaminated items. Clean items are placed on paper towels. Hands are washed when contaminated. Bagging linens, equipment, and garbage is necessary before leaving the room. (TNA 196–199; LTCA 144–146)

6. **D** The first step when putting on a gown is to make sure the gown completely covers your uniform. Tying the strings at the back of neck is the second step. The third step is to overlap the back of the gown. The last step is to tie the waist strings at the back. (TNA 196–199; LTCA 144–146)

7. **C** When removing the gown, untie the waist strings first. Untying the neck strings is the second step. The third step is to pull the gown down from the shoulders. The last step is to wash your hands. (TNA 196–199; LTCA 144–146)

8. **D** Universal precautions are used for all residents regardless of diagnosis. (TNA 192; LTCA 143)

9. **D** Infection precautions are those practices that limit the spread of pathogens. Barriers are set up that prevent the escape of the pathogens, keeping them within a specific area. Pathogens are not destroyed by infection precautions. Nonpathogens are not destroyed by infection precautions. (TNA 192; LTCA 142–143)

10. **C** Biohazardous waste consists of items that are contaminated with the resident's blood, body fluids, or body substances that may be harmful to others. Normal trash consists of items such as newspapers, paper, magazines, etc. Normal waste is another term for normal trash. Biodegradable waste consists of products that break down in landfills with exposure to the sun. (TNA 202; LTCA 150)

CHAPTER 6
The person's comfort
The Patient/Resident Unit
(pp. 37–39)

1. **D** The best solution would be to move the resident to a draft-free location. There is no need to return the resident to bed. Since a lap robe only covers the legs, the resident would still feel a draft over the shoulders. You may not close off a vent without being told to do so. (TNA 253–254; LTCA 194)

2. **D** OBRA requires that nursing facilities maintain a temperature of 71° to 81° F. A temperature range of 68° to 74° F is comfortable for most healthy people. The elderly and chronically ill need higher room temperatures for comfort. To maintain a comfortable working environment for the staff, the temperature should not be higher than 72° to 74° F. Some residents will need extra blankets or clothing for comfort. (TNA 253–254; LTCA 194)

3. **A** People usually relax and rest better in dim light. Soft or natural sunlight may interfere with rest because of glares and shadows. Very bright, cheerful light is stimulating. (TNA 254; LTCA 195–196)

4. **D** Playing music over the intercom increases noise levels. Answering the intercom promptly, speaking quietly, and handling equipment carefully are ways to reduce noise. (TNA 254; LTCA 194–195)

5. **B** The center crank adjusts the bed frame level. The left crank adjusts the head of the bed. The right crank adjusts the knee portion. Side controls are only on electric beds. (TNA 255–256; LTCA 196–199)

6. **D** Only clean or sterile items are placed on the overbed table. It is a working surface for meals, reading, and writing. (LTCA 200; TNA 257)

7. **D** Reverse Trendelenburg's position is where the head of the bed is elevated on blocks and the foot is lowered. Fowler's and semi-Fowler's positions are sitting or semi-sitting positions. Trendelenburg's position is where the foot of the bed is elevated on blocks and the head is lowered. (TNA 256; LTCA 198–199)

Body Mechanics
(pp. 39–41)

1. **C** The back muscles are weak and small. Using the back muscles to lift will often cause back strain. The shoulder, hip, thigh, and upper arm muscles are stronger and larger. (TNA 213; LTCA 158–159)

2. **A** You should not lift a very heavy object. It is best to push, pull, or slide it. (TNA 213; LTCA 158–159)

3. **A** Having the bed as flat as possible enables you to move the resident without resistance. Raising the foot or head of the bed is usually not necessary. The bed should be in a high, working level. (TNA 218–226; LTCA 160–173)

4. **D** With a person on each side of the bed, the resident's weight can be shared evenly. The movement will be smooth and quick. (TNA 224–225; LTCA 166)

5. **D** Grasping the turning sheet at the resident's shoulders and buttocks distributes the weight evenly. This enables you to move the resident in a balanced, smooth movement. Grasping the sheet at other places will result in an unbalanced movement. (TNA 226–227; LTCA 167)

6. **A** The opposite side rail must be up. Having the side rail up on your side makes it difficult for you to move the resident and results in poor body mechanics. The resident's arms are crossed over the chest. Moving the resident to the side of the bed begins at the head and neck and moving downward. You need to stand on the same side of the bed as the resident will be turned to minimize reaching and promote good body mechanics. (TNA 228–229; LTCA 168–169)

7. **D** Logrolling involves turning the resident in one motion, not in segments, to prevent damage to the spine. A mechanical lift is not used. A turning sheet is not always used. (TNA 232; LTCA 173)

8. **C** To distribute the resident's weight evenly, place one of your arms under the shoulders and one under the thighs. (TNA 223–224; LTCA 164–165)

9. **D** Residents on stretchers are never left unattended. Safety straps are always used. The resident is moved feet first. This allows the attendant at the head to watch the resident's breathing and color. Even with the safety straps in place, residents on stretchers are not left alone. (TNA 245; LTCA 185)

10. **C** Three persons are needed to safely transfer a resident on a stretcher to the bed. Two persons are on the opposite side of the stretcher. The third person is on the far side of the bed. (TNA 245; LTCA 185)

11. **B** Transfer belts are applied around the person's waist over clothing. The belt is tightened so it is snug. The buckle is placed either off center in the front or in the back. The belt should not cause discomfort or impair breathing. (TNA 237–241; LTCA 176–181)

12. **D** The resident should get out of bed on the stronger side. This provides some stability to the move. The stronger side helps pull the weaker side along. (TNA 237–241; LTCA 176–181)

13. **A** When a resident cannot tolerate dangling, return him or her to the lying position as quickly as possible. Then report your findings to the nurse. Taking a few deep breaths may not be possible if the resident is having difficulty breathing. Having the resident push both fists into the mattress helps support the sitting position. (TNA 237–241; LTCA 176–181)

14. **D** Dorsal recumbent and supine are the back-lying position. Sims' position is a side-lying position. Prone means lying on the abdomen. Fowler's position is a semi-sitting position. (TNA 247–249; LTCA 186–188)

15. **B** Pillows are not placed under the lower legs in the lateral position. Pillows are placed under the head and shoulders, under the upper legs and thighs, and against the back. (TNA 247–249; LTCA 186–188)

16. **B** For good alignment, the calves should be slightly away from the chair. Feet need to be flat on the floor. The back and buttocks should touch the chair. The backs of the knees need to be slightly away from the seat. (TNA 249; LTCA 189)

Bedmaking
(p. 42)

1. **A** An open bed with the top linens folded back is ready for the resident. Linens are not folded back for a closed bed. A surgical bed has linens folded to one side. An occupied bed refers to making a bed with the resident in it. (TNA 265; LTCA 210)

2. **A** Linens are rolled away from you so that the side that touched the resident is on the inside. Never shake linens or pillows, since shaking them causes the spread of microbes. Never place linen on the floor. This prevents the spread of microbes. Always keep linens away from your uniform. Your uniform is considered dirty. (TNA 266–267; LTCA 212–213)

3. **C** Leftover linen is considered contaminated and cannot be used for other residents. Dirty linen is placed in special bags or hampers. The bottom linen must be wrinkle-free and tight. Make as much of one side of the bed as possible before going to the other side of the bed. This saves energy and time. (TNA 266–267; LTCA 212–213)

4. **B** Collecting linen in the order it will be placed on the bed saves time. Linen rooms may be arranged in several ways. Gather only as much linen as is needed. Select the linens in order. Then turn the stack over to free the arm that had been holding the linens. (TNA 266–267; LTCA 212–213)

5. **B** A closed bed keeps linens clean and wrinkle-free. Open, occupied, or surgical beds are not used for residents who are up most of the day. (TNA 268–270; LTCA 214–215)

6. **C** Plastic drawsheets decrease the resident's comfort because they cause heavy perspiration. Plastic drawsheets do protect the mattress and bottom linens, but can cause discomfort. They increase the risk of skin breakdown. (TNA 266–267; LTCA 212–213)

7. **C** The rules of medical asepsis are followed when making a bed. Medical asepsis consists of the techniques and practices used to keep an area free of pathogens. Surgical asepsis consists of the techniques and practices to keep an area free of pathogens and nonpathogens. Sterile technique consists of the practices used to keep the area free of pathogens and non-pathogens. Isolation procedures are used to prevent the spread of pathogens from one area to another. (TNA 266–267; LTCA 212–213)

8. **D** The linens are considered contaminated and must be put in the dirty laundry. Once linens have been taken into a resident's room they cannot be placed back onto the linen cart. The linen cannot be used for the resident's roommate. The linens cannot go into another room because of the risk of cross contamination. The resulting infection would not save money. (TNA 266–267; LTCA 212–213)

9. **A** When making an occupied bed, the bottom linens are tucked under the resident and then the resident is rolled over the "bump" of linen to the other side. Changing the bed from the top down is occasionally done for persons in traction. The resident does not get up for an occupied bed. Mechanical lifts may be used to help make the bed, but it would then be considered an unoccupied bed. (TNA 274–275; LTCA 219–220)

10. **A** Top linen is mitered at the foot of the bed, but never tucked in on the side. The top sheet is turned down over the blanket. The open end of the pillow is away from the door. The signal light is placed on the bed within the resident's reach. (TNA 269–270; LTCA 214–215)

CHAPTER 7
Cleanliness and skin care
Oral Hygiene
(p. 46)

1. **D** Soft- or medium-bristled toothbrushes are recommended for oral hygiene. Dental floss, toothpaste, and mouthwash are all used to give mouth care. (TNA 285–290; LTCA 231–235)

2. **A** A pink tongue is normal. Cracked lips and swollen and bleeding gums are abnormal. (TNA 285–290; LTCA 231–235)

3. **C** Unconscious residents usually cannot swallow. To protect from aspiration and choking, position the resident on one side. Any other position would be dangerous during mouth care. (TNA 290–292; LTCA 236–237)

4. **C** A padded tongue blade can safely keep the mouth open. Unconscious residents may be able to bite, so never use your fingers. A wash-cloth is too large and makes it difficult to give care. Toothettes or applicators could be bitten and broken. (TNA 290–292; LTCA 236–237)

5. **A** Mouth care is done to keep the mouth moist. Mouth care is done to prevent infections, mouth odors, and to make food taste better. (TNA 285–290; LTCA 231–235)

6. **A** Mouth care on unconscious residents is usually done every 2 hours when the resident is turned and positioned. (TNA 290–292; LTCA 236–237)

7. **C** To reach food and debris, it is necessary to floss below the gums. Flossing more than once a day is a personal choice. All teeth are included in the flossing technique. Rinsing the mouth afterward is helpful. (TNA 285–290; LTCA 231–235)

8. **D** Dentures are brittle and costly and could shatter if dropped in a sink. Care must be taken when cleaning them. Using a towel-lined basin filled with water is a safe method. Holding them firmly with both hands would prevent you from cleaning them. Emesis basins are not big enough. (TNA 292–294; LTCA 238–239)

9. **D** Dentures are cleaned with toothpaste or denture cleaner. Hot water can cause them to warp. Antiseptic mouthwash does not clean dentures completely. Dentures are not flossed. (TNA 292–294; LTCA 238–239)

10. **A** Choking and aspirating are the most serious risks involved in giving mouth care to unconscious residents. Eating toothpaste, talking during the procedure, and biting down on the toothbrush do not involve risk. (TNA 290–292; LTCA 236–237)

Bathing
(pp. 47–48)

1. **D** Whenever possible, the resident's personal preferences should be honored. Baths can be given whenever it is convenient for the resident and the staff. (TNA 295–305; LTCA 240–253)

2. **B** A partial bath cleanses those areas that may develop odors or cause discomfort if not cleansed. The legs and feet are generally not included in the partial bath. The genital area, face, hands, back, and buttocks are washed. (TNA 295–305; LTCA 240–253)

3. **D** Cream and lotion protect the skin from the drying effect of air and evaporation. Soap cleanses the skin, but is drying. Powders absorb moisture and help reduce friction. Deodorants mask and control body odors. (TNA 295–305; LTCA 240–253)

4. **D** Chilling and exposure need to be avoided during any bath. Protecting the resident's privacy and stopping drafts is important. Not all

baths require soap. Always bathe from the cleanest to the dirtiest areas. The nurse decides what type of bath the resident needs. (TNA 295–305; LTCA 240–253)

5. **D** HS care is given to residents at bedtime to help promote comfort and relaxation. It does help increase circulation with the back massage, but this also promotes the resident's comfort and is relaxing. Body and breath odors are prevented, which promotes the resident's comfort. Cleanliness and skin care promote the resident's comfort. (TNA 295–305; LTCA 240–253)

6. **D** Water in the bath basin should be hot (110° to 115° F) because it cools rapidly as it sits. Temperatures below this level would cool too quickly and would be uncomfortable for the resident. (TNA 295–305; LTCA 240–253)

7. **B** Wash from the cleanest to the dirtiest areas. The skin is patted dry to avoid irritating or breaking the skin. The skin should be rinsed thoroughly to prevent dryness. The resident should be covered to provide warmth and privacy. (TNA 295–305; LTCA 240–253)

8. **A** Falling in a slippery, wet shower is a risk for anyone. Special precautions are needed for the elderly. Infection, fainting, and aspiration (choking) are less likely to occur. (TNA 295–305; LTCA 240–253)

9. **C** A tub bath can make a person feel faint, weak, or tired. The water temperature drops and causes chilling if the bath does not end in 20 minutes. (TNA 295–305; LTCA 240–253)

10. **C** A shower chair allows the resident to sit during the shower. Water drains through an opening in the seat. Bath mats help prevent slipping but are of little use if the resident cannot stand. Wheelchairs are not plastic and should not be used in showers. A mechanical lift is used to lift residents into a tub. (TNA 295–305; LTCA 240–253)

11. **B** The body is always bathed from the cleanest to the dirtiest areas. The bath always begins with the face. Washing the far arm first, then the near arm, prevents water from dripping on areas already cleaned. The chest is washed after the arms. (TNA 295–305; LTCA 240–253)

12. **B** The urethra is the cleanest part of the perineal area. The anal area is the dirtiest. Washing from the urethra to the anal area follows medical asepsis and washing from the cleanest to the dirtiest areas. (TNA 295–305; LTCA 240–253)

13. **A** The tip of the penis is cleaned using a circular motion starting at the urethral opening. The shaft of the penis is washed with firm, downward strokes. The anal area is the last part to be cleaned in perineal care. Uncircumcised males need to have the foreskin retracted. (TNA 308–310; LTCA 256–259)

14. **C** The anal area is cleaned by wiping from the woman's vagina to the anus, then discarding the washcloth. Gloves are used. Since the area is very sensitive, warm (not hot) water is used. Cleaning from front to back in one stroke follows the rules of medical asepsis. (TNA 308–310; LTCA 256–259)

15. **C** Residents prefer to do their own perineal care. It is embarrassing to have it done by others. Independence is not a major reason for letting residents do their own perineal care. Residents may or may not perform this care more frequently. The care can be done equally as well by the staff as by the resident. (TNA 308–310; LTCA 256–259)

16. **A** Locking shower chair wheels stabilizes the chair for the shower. Leaving them unlocked does not. Shower chairs are designed to be used in water. There is no need to cover the wheels with plastic. Rusting is not a problem. (TNA 295–305; LTCA 240–253)

17. **A** This observation is reported to the nurse. Rubbing the area vigorously with the lotion can cause the area to break down even more. Checking the area again is important, but only after it has been reported. The nurse decides what care needs to be given. (TNA 312–317; LTCA 276–280)

18. **A** Making a mitt prevents the loose ends of the washcloth from dragging across the resident. Folding the washcloth into fourths or holding it like a ball or sponge does not give you the neat, efficient grasp of the mitt. (TNA 299; LTCA 243)

19. **D** Bath water is changed frequently during the bath. It is changed when it becomes cold, soapy, after washing the feet, and before giving perineal care. The doors and windows are closed to avoid drafts and provide privacy. Bath blankets are warmer and more comfortable for residents than are sheets. If possible, residents should perform their own perineal care. (TNA 295–305; LTCA 240–253)

20. **C** Patting the skin dry is less irritating than rubbing it. Lotion is often used to protect dry skin. Residents with dry, fragile skin may not get complete baths daily. While soap use should be limited, it is needed to cleanse the skin, which should be rinsed well. Water temperature of 100° F is too cool for bathing. (TNA 295–305; LTCA 240–253)

Dressing and Grooming
(pp. 50–51)

1. **A** It is important to clean the face before shaving. This reduces the amount of bacteria on the skin. Applying lather and shaving in the direction of the hair growth are later steps in the procedure. After washing the face, apply a wet

washcloth or towel to the face to soften the beard. (TNA 326–327; LTCA 264–265)

2. **C** Braiding keeps the hair from tangling. This can only be done with the resident's permission. Oiling the hair will not prevent tangling. Cutting the hair is not allowed. Shampooing the hair will not prevent tangling. (TNA 321–325; LTCA 260–263)

3. **A** Since the right arm is paralyzed, first remove the gown from the left (unaffected) arm. Starting with the right arm is incorrect and would be very difficult. Turning the resident on the left side prevents you from removing the gown. A clean garment is put on after the soiled garment is removed. (TNA 330–340; LTCA 268–275)

4. **C** When there is an IV, the gown is removed from the unaffected arm first. Never cut the sleeve. If you begin with the arm with the IV, it will be awkward to remove the gown. **NEVER** disconnect IV tubing! (TNA 330–340; LTCA 268–275)

5. **B** Hair is brushed from the scalp to the hair ends to distribute the oils from the scalp along the hair shaft. Begin at the top of the head on one side. Remove the resident's eyeglasses so you do not accidentally pull off the glasses while brushing. Brush with downward, not upward strokes. (TNA 321–325; LTCA 260–263)

6. **D** A washcloth or hand towel is used to shield the resident's eyes from water and shampoo. It must be over the eyes, not over the nose and mouth. That could interfere with breathing. Use both hands to apply lather. Massage the scalp gently with the fingertips. Water should be at a temperature of 110° F. (TNA 321–325; LTCA 260–263)

7. **A** You should not shampoo a resident's hair unless the nurse tells you to. Some facilities have a beautician. It is the nurse's job to arrange this, if possible. Brushing and combing do not take the place of shampooing. (TNA 321–325; LTCA 260–263)

8. **B** Minor bleeding is easily stopped by applying direct pressure. Aftershave lotion causes discomfort when applied to open skin. Bandages are not necessary for small nicked areas. The area may continue to bleed if pressure is not applied. (TNA 326–327; LTCA 264–265)

9. **C** A hand-held nozzle is not essential. When shampooing in bed, water is poured over the hair with a pitcher. The shampoo and trough are essential items. (TNA 321–325; LTCA 260–263)

10. **B** Nursing assistants do not trim toenails. Nails are cut straight across. Soaking the nails helps soften them for cutting. Clippers are used to trim fingernails. (TNA 328–329; LTCA 266–267)

Back Massage
(p. 52)

1. **A** A back massage is given to relax muscles and stimulate circulation. Muscles are not exercised. (TNA 306–307; LTCA 254–255)

2. **B** The back rub should last 3 to 5 minutes. This gives time to work all areas of the back and shoulders. Ten minutes or more is unreasonable. (TNA 306–307; LTCA 254–255)

3. **B** Lotion is used to reduce friction during the back massage. Soap dries the skin. Bath oil is too messy and greasy. Rubbing alcohol cools and dries the skin. (TNA 306–307; LTCA 254–255)

4. **A** With the resident in the prone position, all areas of the back and shoulders can be massaged. The supine and Fowler's positions do not allow contact with the back area. The side-lying position is acceptable, but it prevents massaging some parts of the back. (TNA 306–307; LTCA 254–255)

5. **D** The back massage should end with long, firm movements. Circular motions are used over bony parts. Kneading and fast movements are done during the massage. (TNA 306–307; LTCA 254–255)

CHAPTER 8
Elimination
Maintaining Normal Elimination
(pp. 53–54)

1. **C** Particles in the urine need to be reported. Normal urine is pale yellow, clear, and has a faint ammonia odor. (TNA 343–352; LTCA 286–306)

2. **B** Top linens are folded back out of the way. They do not need to be removed. They are not changed unless they are wet or soiled. A bath blanket is not necessary. (TNA 343–352; LTCA 286–306)

3. **D** Fracture pans have a thinner rim. They are more comfortable for residents with limited range of motion. Residents must get out of bed to use commodes. Catheters are only used by the nurses with a doctor's order. Urinals are used by male residents. (TNA 343–352; LTCA 286–306)

4. **D** This method does not require the resident to assist. Lifting the buttocks should not be attempted alone. Turning the resident toward you is incorrect body mechanics. Family members may offer to help but should not be expected to do so. (TNA 343–352; LTCA 286–306)

5. **B** It is best to leave the room and give the resident privacy. If you must stay with the resident, remain nearby. Do not sit or stand at the bedside. Doing tasks in the room may be distracting. (TNA 343–352; LTCA 286–306)

6. **D** If residents cannot wipe after urinating, you must do this for them. Toilet tissue is used, not cotton balls. A partial bath is usually not necessary. It is not necessary to report this. (TNA 343–352; LTCA 286–306)

7. **B** Men prefer to urinate standing up. Sitting or lying down can interfere with urination in men. (TNA 343–352; LTCA 286–306)

8. **C** You do not need to soak bedpans in disinfectant. Cover bedpans when taking them to dispose of contents. Always rinse them with water. Use a disinfectant as directed (often a spray). Return bedpans to bedside stands. (TNA 343–352; LTCA 286–306)

9. **D** Commodes are chair-like and are used at the bedside. They cannot be used for bedridden residents. (TNA 343–352; LTCA 286–306)

10. **B** Whenever residents urinate, allow them to wash their hands. Nursing assistants measure the urine, not the resident. Residents may or may not return to bed after using commodes. It is not necessary to call the nurse unless there is a problem. (TNA 343–352; LTCA 286–306)

11. **B** Voiding small amounts frequently must be reported. It is normal to void before meals, at bedtime, and upon awakening. Males prefer to stand to void. Voiding 250 ml every 5 hours is normal. (TNA 343–352; LTCA 286–306)

12. **A** Fowler's position lets the resident sit on the bedpan. This is the normal position. Prone and side-lying positions make it impossible to use the bedpan. The supine position puts stress on the lower back. The head of the bed needs to be raised slightly. (TNA 343–352; LTCA 286–306)

Catheters
(p. 55)

1. **D** Retention and indwelling are other terms for a Foley catheter. The other responses are made-up terms. (TNA 352–358; LTCA 294–299)

2. **C** The nurse inflates a small balloon at the tip of the catheter after insertion. This prevents the catheter from slipping out. Taping prevents the tubing from irritating the meatus. Neither muscles nor positioning would keep a catheter in place. (TNA 352–358; LTCA 294–299)

3. **C** The collection bag is attached to the bed frame so the bag remains below the level of the bladder. It would be uncomfortable if attached to the resident's leg. There is no way to attach the bag to the mattress. The side rails are moved too frequently and would pull on the catheter tubing. (TNA 352–358; LTCA 294–299)

4. **D** The collection bag can easily hold the amount of urine passed in an 8-hour period.

This also allows for accurate record keeping. The bag must be emptied more than once a day. (TNA 352–358; LTCA 294–299)

5. **D** Always keep the collection bag below the level of the bladder. This prevents the urine from flowing back into the urethra and bladder. Tubing should be coiled on the bed without kinks so that the urine flows freely. The catheter is taped to the resident's thigh. (TNA 352–358; LTCA 294–299)

6. **B** Observation is a first step in procedures. Applying antiseptic solution, cleaning the catheter, and taping it properly are steps that follow. (TNA 352–358; LTCA 294–299)

7. **B** The tubing is **never** disconnected from the bag. This allows bacteria to enter the system. The catheter and urinary drainage bag are considered a "closed system." The other steps are part of the procedure. (TNA 352–358; LTCA 294–299)

8. **C** Clamping a catheter lets urine collect in the bladder. This helps restore muscle tone. Bladder training begins by clamping for short periods (such as an hour), then longer periods. The catheter remains in for a period of time. The resident will not use the toilet until the catheter is removed. (TNA 352–358; LTCA 294–299)

9. **C** The inability to control the passage of urine from the bladder is called urinary incontinence. Catheterization is the process of inserting a catheter. Elimination means removing waste from the body. Involuntary urination is not a recognized term. (TNA 343; LTCA 285)

10. **C** Infection is the greatest risk from an indwelling catheter. Pain and bleeding usually do not occur. (TNA 352–358; LTCA 294–299)

Collecting and Testing Urine Specimens
(p. 56)

1. **A** When collecting a urine specimen, you need to use the appropriate container. The container needs to be accurately labeled with the requested information. The specimen needs to be collected at the specified time and taken to the lab or designated area. (TNA 359–367; LTCA 300–305)

2. **D** A double-voided urine specimen is called a fresh-fractional urine specimen. (TNA 359–367; LTCA 300–305)

3. **C** 24-hour specimens must be kept cold. Urine strainers are used when kidney stones are suspected. Antiseptic solution is not used with urine samples. Testape is used to check urine for sugar. (TNA 359–367; LTCA 300–305)

4. **A** There are no restrictions for routine urine specimens. (TNA 359–367; LTCA 300–305)

5. **C** Perineal care reduces the number of microorganisms in the urethral area when the specimen is obtained. The other points refer to other tests. (TNA 359–367; LTCA 300–305)

6. **B** The bladder is emptied of "stale" urine. "Fresh" urine produced in 30 minutes is used to test for sugar. Large amounts of urine are not needed. A sterile specimen is not required. (TNA 359–367; LTCA 300–305)

7. **D** A 24-hour urine specimen involves collecting all urine voided by a resident during a 24-hour period. (TNA 359–367; LTCA 300–305)

8. **A** When collecting a 24-hour urine specimen, you should discard the first voiding. (TNA 359–367; LTCA 300–305)

9. **B** Do not touch the inside of the container. The sample must be free of toilet tissue. It must be properly labeled. A clean container is used for each sample. (TNA 359–367; LTCA 300–305)

10. **A** When you find a stone in the resident's urine, you should take the stone to the nurse. It will be sent to the laboratory to be examined. (TNA 359–367; LTCA 300–305)

Bowel Elimination
(pp. 57–58)

1. **B** Feces are normally brown and soft-formed. Some people have bowel movements every day, others every 2 or 3 days. Defecation can occur at any time. (TNA 371–372; LTCA 310–311)

2. **C** Diarrhea occurs when feces travel through the intestine very rapidly. This prevents the colon from absorbing water. The stool is very soft, formed stools. (TNA 375–376; LTCA 312)

3. **B** Peristalsis slows with aging. Factors such as illness and medication can affect elimination. Exercise and certain foods stimulate peristalsis. (TNA 372; LTCA 311)

4. **D** Enemas are only given when ordered by the doctor. Many other measures can be taken for the resident who has difficulty having a bowel movement. Enemas may be ordered before certain x-ray films are taken. Fluid is introduced into the rectum and colon for an enema. (TNA 376–384; LTCA 313–319)

5. **D** The opening surgically created between the colon and the abdomen is called a colostomy. An ileostomy involves the small bowel. The opening is called a stoma. The surgical creation of an opening is called an ostomy. (TNA 386–388; LTCA 321–323)

6. **B** With an ileostomy, the stool consistency will be liquid. Because the entire colon has been removed, fecal material is liquid. Water cannot be absorbed. Neither the resident's diet nor age will affect this. (TNA 386–388; LTCA 321–323)

7. **B** A rectal tube is inserted 2 to 4 inches beyond the anal opening. The tube must be in the rectum to function. Injury to the intestinal wall can occur if the tube is passed beyond 4 inches. (TNA 385–386; LTCA 320)

8. **C** An enema solution should be 105° F. Cooler solution can be uncomfortable and less effective. Warmer solution can damage the delicate lining of the colon. (TNA 376–384; LTCA 313–319)

9. **C** Raising the fluid above the level of the resident increases pressure and forces fluid into the colon. If not raised at least 18 inches above the mattress (12 inches above the anus), fluid may not enter into the rectum. If the bag is raised higher, cramping and difficulty in retaining the fluid can occur. (TNA 376–384; LTCA 313–319)

10. **B** The traditional enema position is the left Sims' position. The elderly often prefer a left side-lying position. This lets enema solution flow more easily into the bowel. (TNA 376–384; LTCA 313–319)

11. **B** Rectal tubes are used to relieve flatulence without effort from the intestine. It is not meant to remove stool. (TNA 385–386; LTCA 320)

12. **D** An oil-retention enema is given to relieve constipation or fecal impaction. These types of stools are very hard and may be large and difficult to pass. Oil is retained and softens the stool, which allows for easy passage. (TNA 376–384; LTCA 313–319)

13. **C** A tongue blade is used to transfer a stool specimen from the bedpan to the specimen container because it is disposable. A spoon or alcohol wipes are not appropriate. Applicators are too small. (TNA 391–394; LTCA 326–327)

14. **B** Stool specimens must be free of urine for an accurate test. Medical asepsis rules are followed. Some samples are kept warm. Two tablespoons are enough for a sample. (TNA 391–394; LTCA 326–327)

15. **C** Reusable appliances are cleaned with soap and water and allowed to dry. They are not sent to the laundry or cleaned by the family. Heat in the autoclave would cause melting. (TNA 386–388; LTCA 321–323)

16. **C** Skin around the stoma needs special attention. Use warm water and soap (only if ordered) to clean the skin. All other agents are too harsh. (TNA 386–388; LTCA 321–323)

17. **D** Colostomy appliances are changed whenever soiling occurs. This varies greatly from person to person. (TNA 386–388; LTCA 321–323)

18. **A** Because of the liquid consistency, the ileostomy drains all the time. (TNA 386–388; LTCA 321–323)

19. **D** Ileostomy appliances are sealed to the skin and remain in place for 2 to 4 days. A prescribed

solvent is needed for appliance removal. Alcohol, water, and Karaya powder will not remove it properly. (TNA 386–388; LTCA 321–323)

20. **C** Colostomy appliances are disposable and not reused. A new bag is used. Avoiding gas-forming foods can reduce colostomy odors. Good hygiene is essential. Deodorants can help. (TNA 386–388; LTCA 321–323)

CHAPTER 9
Foods and fluids
Foods and Fluids
(pp. 61–63)

1. **D** The main nutrients in milk are protein, calcium, fat, carbohydrates, and riboflavin. (TNA 397–407; LTCA 332–338)

2. **C** Adults need 6 to 11 servings from the bread and cereal group a day. (TNA 397–407; LTCA 332–338)

3. **B** Citrus fruits are one of the best sources of vitamin C. Liver is high in vitamins A, D, and K. When skin is exposed to sunlight, it provides a source of vitamin D. Fish liver oils contain vitamin D. (TNA 397–407; LTCA 332–338)

4. **B** Vitamins A, D, E, and K are stored by the body. They are commonly obtained through food. Vitamins have no caloric value. The body cannot produce vitamins. (TNA 397–407; LTCA 332–338)

5. **A** A serving of meat or fish is 2 to 3 ounces. This is far smaller than what most people actually believe to be a "serving." (TNA 397–407; LTCA 332–338)

6. **D** Between-meal nourishments are served when they arrive on the nursing unit. These nourishments are part of the therapeutic diet plan. Residents must receive them on time. (TNA 419; LTCA 349)

7. **C** Edema means swelling. It has little to do with the appetite. It is the opposite of dehydration. (TNA 397; LTCA 331)

8. **C** The resident should be allowed to choose the order in which the food is eaten. This respects the dignity and independence of the resident. (TNA 417; LTCA 348)

9. **A** Using the numbers of a clock as areas on the tray is an easy way for a blind resident to locate food. Touching, smelling, or tasting does not help the resident locate food on the tray. (TNA 418; LTCA 349)

10. **B** NPO means nothing by mouth. All of the other residents can and should have drinking water. (TNA 419; LTCA 350)

11. **A** A graduate is calibrated in milliliters or cubic centimeters. This insures consistency in all measurements. An emesis basin, water pitcher, or measuring cup are not calibrated finely enough. (TNA 413; LTCA 343)

12. **B** Calories are taken into account in diabetic diets. The timing of meals is very important. Carbohydrates as well as fat and proteins are controlled. Only the food allowed and all food served should be eaten. (TNA 410; LTCA 341)

13. **C** Ice cream is high in fat. Bread, skim milk, and potatoes are low in fat and are allowed on low-cholesterol diets. (TNA 397–407; LTCA 332–338)

14. **A** Unless the gown is soiled, there is no need to change it. Allowing voiding, offering oral hygiene, and helping the resident to a comfortable position are necessary. (TNA 417; LTCA 347)

15. **C** 2000 to 2500 ml of fluid are required for an adult to maintain normal fluid balance. 1500 ml allows survival. Less than 1500 ml is not considered an adequate fluid intake. (TNA 412–413; LTCA 342–343)

16. **B** These items are nearly impossible to measure. Ounce equivalencies are available for gelatin, popsicles, creamed cereals, ice cream, sherbet, custard, and pudding. (TNA 413; LTCA 343)

17. **C** 150 ml. Graduates are calibrated in ounces and milliliters. Intake is usually measured in milliliters (ml) or cubic centimeters (cc). (TNA 415; LTCA 343)

18. **D** 350 cc. Milliliters and cubic centimeters are equal. (TNA 415; LTCA 343)

CHAPTER 10
Vital signs
Measurement of Vital Signs
(pp. 65–67)

1. **C** Bowel function is not measured for vital signs. Only heart function, respirations, and body temperature are included because they reflect the three body processes essential for life: regulation of body temperature, breathing, and heart function. (TNA 427; LTCA 358)

2. **C** The sphygmomanometer and stethoscope are used to measure blood pressure. A watch is needed to time the counting of the pulse and respirations. A thermometer is used for temperature. (TNA 450–453; LTCA 379–381)

3. **D** Body temperature rises with activity. An early morning temperature is usually the lowest of the day. The temperature rises slightly with activity and meals. (TNA 428–440; LTCA 358–371)

4. **D** A normal oral temperature should not exceed 99.6° F. Axillary temperatures should not exceed 98.6° F. Rectal temperatures above 100.6° F should be reported. (TNA 428–440; LTCA 358–371)

5. **C** A rectal temperature is inserted only 1 inch into the rectum. For accurate readings, glass thermometers are held in place for at least 2 minutes. The tip must be lubricated. A glass thermometer must always be shaken down before use. (TNA 428–440; LTCA 358–371)

6. **D** Glass thermometers are washed in cold, soapy water for cleaning. Some facilities store glass thermometers in a disinfectant. Wiping the glass thermometer with alcohol will not sufficiently clean it. Wiping with a tissue only removes excess mucus or fecal material. This does not clean the thermometer. Hot water causes the mercury to climb, which could break the thermometer. (TNA 428–440; LTCA 358–371)

7. **A** Electronic thermometers register accurate temperatures in 2 to 60 seconds. A glass thermometer takes 2 to 3 minutes for an oral temperature, at least 2 minutes for a rectal temperature, and 5 to 10 minutes for an axillary temperature. Tympanic membrane sensors measure temperatures in 1 to 3 seconds. (TNA 428–440; LTCA 358–371)

8. **D** Axillary temperatures should range from 96.6° to 98.6° F, or 36° to 37° C. (TNA 428–440; LTCA 358–371)

9. **B** Residents receiving oxygen by mask should not have the oxygen interrupted. Therefore the oral temperature is not taken. The oral route is used for alert and cooperative residents and for those with heart disease or diarrhea. (TNA 428–440; LTCA 358–371)

10. **A** The oral thermometer is placed under the tongue close to superficial blood vessels. This gives a small, pocket-like area for accurate temperature measurement. Other locations in the mouth would register lower, inaccurate readings. (TNA 428–440; LTCA 358–371)

11. **D** The adult pulse rate is between 60 and 100 beats per minute. A pulse rate of 120 beats per minute would need to be reported to the nurse immediately; it exceeds the normal range for pulse rates. (TNA 440–447; LTCA 371–377)

12. **B** The radial pulse is the site usually used for measuring a pulse. Apical pulses are taken on residents who have heart disease or who are taking medication that affects the heart. The brachial pulse is used to measure blood pressure. The femoral pulse is not usually used to take a pulse. (TNA 440–447; LTCA 371–377)

13. **C** If the pulse is irregular, it is counted for 1 full minute. The pulse is felt by placing the first three fingers of one hand against the radial pulse. Do not use your thumb to take a pulse; it has a pulse of its own. The pulse is counted for 30 seconds and multiplied by 2. The pulse may be strong, full, or bounding, and sometimes it is thready and hard to find. (TNA 440–447; LTCA 371–377)

14. **D** A hard-to-feel pulse is described as being weak and thready. Full and bounding describes a strong, forceful pulse. Irregular and regular describes the rhythm, not the quality or force. (TNA 440–447; LTCA 371–377)

15. **D** Since stethoscopes are often shared by various workers, the chances of cross contamination are great. The earpieces and diaphragm are cleaned with alcohol before and after each use. Alcohol wipes are a handy form of disinfectant. Earpieces are not disposable. Soap and water could damage the stethoscope. A stethoscope cannot be sterilized. (TNA 440–447; LTCA 371–377)

16. **A** An apical pulse is counted for 1 full minute. One minute lets the listener hear the pattern of the heartbeat and the rate. An irregular pattern may be missed with less time. (TNA 440–447; LTCA 371–377)

17. **C** The apical pulse is located on the left side of the chest, below the nipple line. The radial pulse is on the thumb side of the wrist. The brachial artery is located on the inner aspect of the bend in the elbow. (TNA 440–447; LTCA 371–377)

18. **D** Since respirations can be controlled voluntarily, the resident should not know that you are counting the respirations. Watch or feel the rise and fall of the resident's chest to count the respirations. By continuing to hold the resident's wrist, it appears that the pulse is still being counted. Counting for 30 seconds will let you identify any abnormal patterns. (TNA 448; LTCA 378)

19. **D** Tachypnea means that respirations are greater than 24 per minute. Less than 10 respirations per minute is called bradypnea. Dyspnea is difficult, labored, or painful breathing. Normal respirations are between 10 and 20 breaths per minute. (TNA 448; LTCA 378)

20. **B** Apnea means no breathing. Slow, shallow, and irregular respirations are called hypoventilation. Rapid, deep respirations are known as hyperventilation. (TNA 448; LTCA 378)

21. **C** The normal systolic pressure ranges from 100 to 140 mm Hg. Normal diastolic pressure is 60 to 90 mm Hg. In the elderly, a systolic pressure between 100 and 160 mm Hg and a diastolic pressure of 60 to 95 mm Hg is normal. (TNA 450–453; LTCA 379–381)

22. **B** The brachial artery is used to determine blood pressure. The radial artery is usually used to determine the pulse. The carotid and femoral arteries are not appropriate. (TNA 450–453; LTCA 379–381)

23. **A**   The cuff is applied to the bare upper arm. Clothing can affect the measurement. Blood pressures are not taken in the arm with an IV infusion. The diastolic reading is the point at which the sound disappears. The resident should rest 15 minutes before taking the blood pressure. (TNA 450–453; LTCA 379–381)

24. **A**   The systolic blood pressure is the point where the first sound is heard. The point where the last sound is heard is the diastolic pressure. (TNA 450–453; LTCA 379–381)

25. **D**   Consistently high blood pressure is called hypertension. Heart failure is when the heart weakens. Pulse deficit is the difference in apical and radial pulse rates. Hypotension is low blood pressure. (TNA 450–453; LTCA 379–381)

CHAPTER 11
Exercise, activity, and restorative care
Preventing the Complications of Bed Rest
(pp. 69–70)

1. **C**   The resident on bed rest may be allowed to take part in activities of daily living. What the person may be allowed to do varies from facility to facility. Contractures and muscle atrophy can occur. Bed rest does reduce pain and promotes healing. Serious complications can occur as a result of bed rest. Pressure sores, constipation, and fecal impactions can occur. Blood clots, urinary tract infections, and pneumonia may also occur. (TNA 457; LTCA 386)

2. **D**   Atrophy is the decrease in size or the wasting away of tissue. Once a contracture develops, it is a permanent disability. Contractures are the permanent abnormal shortenings of muscles. ROM exercises help prevent contractures. (TNA 458; LTCA 386)

3. **C**   Bed boards are placed under the mattress to prevent it from sagging. The footboard prevents plantar flexion. A bed cradle and a footboard keep top linens off the feet. Trochanter rolls keep the hips from rotating outwardly. (TNA 458; LTCA 387)

4. **B**   Plantar flexion (footdrop) is prevented by using a footboard. Handrolls are used to prevent contractures of the thumb, fingers, and wrist. A bed cradle and a footboard keep top linens off the feet. Bed boards are placed under the mattress to prevent it from sagging. Trochanter rolls keep the hips from rotating outwardly. (TNA 458; LTCA 387)

5. **D**   External rotation is the outward turning of a joint. Abduction occurs when a body part moves away from the body. Adduction is the movement of a body part toward the body. Internal rotation is the inward turning of a joint. (TNA 460–465; LTCA 386–393)

6. **D**   Trochanter rolls prevent hips and legs from turning outward. A trapeze is used by the resident to lift the trunk of the body off the bed. A footboard keeps the feet in good alignment. Bed cradles keep top linens off of the resident's feet. (TNA 459; LTCA 388)

7. **C**   The weight of linens on the foot can cause footdrop and pressure sores. Bed cradles keep top linens off the resident's feet. A trapeze is used by the resident to lift the trunk of the body off the bed. Bed boards are placed under the mattress to prevent it from sagging. Trochanter rolls prevent hips and legs from turning outward. (TNA 458–459; LTCA 387–388)

8. **C**   The trapeze swings from a bed frame over the resident. It is helpful for exercising, moving and turning in bed, and lifting the trunk off the bed. It does not prevent external rotation of the hip. (TNA 458–460; LTCA 387–389)

9. **C**   Passive range-of-motion exercises are performed by another person for the resident. Active range-of-motion exercises are done by the resident. The nurse will tell you which joints to exercise, the frequency of the exercises, and if the exercises are to be active, passive, or active-assistive. Active-assistive range-of-motion exercise means that the person does the exercises with some assistance from another person. (TNA 460–465; LTCA 386–393)

10. **B**   Adduction means a body part is moved toward the body. Extension is the straightening of a body part. Abduction means going "away from." Supination means "turning upward." (TNA 460–465; LTCA 386–393)

11. **A**   Bending a body part is called flexion. Extension is the straightening of a part. Dorsiflexion means bending backward. Hyperextension is excessive straightening of a body part. (TNA 460–465; LTCA 386–393)

12. **B**   Do not force a joint beyond its present range-of-motion or to the point of pain. (TNA 460–465; LTCA 386–393)

13. **B**   Range-of-motion exercises should be repeated five to six times. (TNA 460–465; LTCA 386–393)

14. **C**   Abduction is to move a body part away from the body. Flexion is bending a body part. Extension is straightening a body part. Adduction is moving a body part toward the body. (TNA 460–465; LTCA 386–393)

15. **A**   Flexion is bending a body part. Extension is straightening a body part. Dorsiflexion is bending a joint backward. Hyperextension is the

excessive straightening of a body part. (TNA 460–465; LTCA 386–393)

Pressure Sores
(pp. 71–72)

1. **D** Plastic drawsheets and waterproof pads are not used because they hold moisture close to the skin. All of the other items are used to treat pressure sores. (TNA 314–317; LTCA 276–280)
2. **A** Bony areas create pressure points when residents lie in bed or sit for long periods of time. Soft, well-padded areas are not subject to this pressure. Pressure sores are different than the ulcers that develop in the mouth or stomach. (TNA 312–314; LTCA 276–277)
3. **B** Pressure and friction are the most common causes of skin to breakdown. These are the most common causes of pressure sores. Moisture or dry skin also contribute but are not the most common causes. Poor circulation to any area contributes to pressure sore formation. Irritation by urine and feces also contributes to skin breakdown. (TNA 312; LTCA 277)
4. **B** Scrubbing and rubbing the skin (especially skin that is dry) can lead to skin breakdown. Repositioning, applying lotion, and keeping the linens fresh are helpful in preventing pressure sores. (TNA 315; LTCA 278)
5. **B** Egg crate mattresses are placed on top of regular mattresses. They are not washable and are discarded when they are soiled. Peaks distribute the resident's weight more evenly. The bottom sheet covers both the egg crate and regular mattress. (TNA 314–317; LTCA 276–280)

Ambulation and Walking Aids
(pp. 72–73)

1. **A** The resident should be encouraged to stand erect with the back straight and head up. This promotes good body alignment and balance. The pace should be set by the resident. The resident should be encouraged to walk normally. Shuffling the feet is discouraged. Walking aids are used when needed or when ordered by the doctor. (TNA 466–472; LTCA 394–402)
2. **C** A walker gives more support than a cane. It is preferred by most residents who need walking aids. Braces support a weak body part, such as the knee or back. Crutches are used when one or both legs need to gain strength. Canes give support and balance when one side of the body is weak. (TNA 466–472; LTCA 394–402)
3. **B** Helping the falling resident to move safely to the floor is the best action. Trying to prevent the fall could cause greater harm. Trying to steady the resident or regain balance may cause the resident and/or the nursing assistant to twist, strain, or injure the head. It would be unreasonable to get the resident back to bed. (TNA 466–472; LTCA 394–402)
4. **D** A single-tipped cane is held on the strong side of the body. The grip should be at hip level. Canes provide balance and support. When walking, the cane is moved first. (TNA 466–472; LTCA 394–402)
5. **A** A walker is moved about 6 inches in front of the resident. Distances greater than 6 inches could cause the resident to lose his/her balance and fall. (TNA 466–472; LTCA 394–402)
6. **D** Braces do not assist with range-of-motion exercises because they prevent joint movement. They support a weak body part. A brace can prevent or correct deformities. (TNA 466–472; LTCA 394–402)

Rehabilitation
(pp. 73–74)

1. **A** Rehabilitation involves the whole person, not just physical disabilities. It stresses physical capabilities and the person's psychological and social function. (TNA 569; LTCA 470)
2. **A** Successful rehabilitation depends on the person's attitude, acceptance of limitations, and motivation. The person must focus on remaining abilities. Sometimes improvement is not possible. Then the focus is on maintaining the highest level of functioning possible and preventing further disability. The person is encouraged to perform as many activities of daily living as possible and to the extent possible. (TNA 569; LTCA 470)
3. **D** Rehabilitation begins the moment a person enters a health care facility. The goal is to prevent complications and to help the person reach the highest level of functioning possible. (TNA 569–579; LTCA 470–478)
4. **A** Anger is a normal response to a disability. The rehabilitative process lets the person express anger in a healthy way. Other complications prevented include pressure ulcers, contractures, and bowel or bladder problems. (TNA 576; LTCA 474)
5. **C** A prosthesis is an artificial body part. Examples of self-help devices are eating utensils with cuffs and glass holders. Examples of methods of rehabilitation would be range-of-motion exercises and bowel training. A suppository is a solid medication that melts at body temperature. (TNA 576; LTCA 474)
6. **B** The rehabilitation team is centered around the resident. (TNA 576; LTCA 474)

7. **D**   Your role is to support, reassure, and encourage the resident. You cannot truthfully say that everything will be okay. Leaving the individual alone only adds to feelings of loneliness, uselessness, and despair. Saying that depression, anger, and hostility "slow down progress" does not help the resident. (TNA 569–579; LTCA 470–478)

CHAPTER 12
Special procedures and treatments
Heat and Cold Applications
(pp. 75–76)

1. **A**   Heat causes the blood vessels to relax and dilate (open wider). Contract, constrict, and become narrow all describe the same action. This is the effect of cold on blood vessels. (TNA 511; LTCA 430)

2. **D**   A moist heat application means that water is in contact with the skin. A complication is an adverse condition that occurs as a result of the treatment. Dry heat means that no moisture or water is in contact with the skin. A local heat application means that heat is applied to a small body area. (TNA 512; LTCA 430)

3. **D**   Heat applications cause an increase in the blood supply to a body part. Pain relief, healing, and relaxation are promoted by heat applications. (TNA 511; LTCA 430)

4. **B**   Burns are the greatest danger of a heat application. Loss of consciousness or central nervous system damage are not likely to occur. Heat causes the blood flow to increase. (TNA 511; LTCA 430)

5. **B**   Water is a good conductor of heat. This means that the effects of the heat are greater and faster than with a dry application. A moist heat application means that water is in contact with the skin. Heat does penetrate more deeply than with a dry heat application. The temperature of the application is lower than that of a dry heat application. (TNA 512; LTCA 430)

6. **D**   Heat can be in contact with the skin too long. This causes the blood vessels to constrict, and reduces blood flow. Because the skin appears pale, it must be reported immediately. Skin is reddened and warm when a heat application is working. Measure the temperature of a heat application for accuracy. Swelling is reduced gradually over a period of time. (TNA 511; LTCA 430)

7. **B**   Hot compresses should remain in place about 20 minutes. The area under the hot compress is checked every 5 minutes for redness and complaints of pain, discomfort, or numbness. Commercial compresses are heated for 10 minutes, or as instructed by the nurse, under an ultraviolet light. Heat applied for more than 1 hour causes blood vessels to constrict and complications to develop. (TNA 512; LTCA 431)

8. **A**   The sitz bath involves immersing the pelvic area in warm or hot water for 20 minutes. The sitz bath increases the blood flow to the pelvic area, thereby reducing the blood flow to other body parts. This relaxing effect may cause the resident to become weak or faint during the procedure. Sitz baths are used to cleanse the perineum, relieve pain, increase circulation, or to stimulate voiding. (TNA 516–517; LTCA 435–436)

9. **D**   Compresses are applied to small parts of the body. They are not used for large areas or the entire body. Bruised, tense, swollen, cold, or painful areas can benefit from this application. (TNA 512–514; LTCA 431–433)

10. **B**   Never cover the lamp because a fire might occur. The lamp is removed after 20 to 30 minutes because it may burn the person. The distance from the bulb to the resident is measured. Stop the treatment immediately if the resident complains of pain, burning, or decreased sensation. (TNA 511–521; LTCA 430–439)

11. **A**   When changing the water, wrap the part in a towel while the water is being changed. Leaving the part in the cool water would be uncomfortable for the resident. The soak should last for the length of time ordered by the physician. Applying a hot compress or aquathermia pad would not be appropriate. (TNA 511–521; LTCA 430–439)

12. **C**   A flannel cover offers a thin, soft layer of protection from the bag. Yet it lets the heat penetrate. A towel is too thick to let heat reach the skin. Covering it with plastic or a bed protector would offer little or no protection. (TNA 511–521; LTCA 430–439)

13. **D**   Once the cover becomes wet, the heat application is considered moist. The risk of burns increases. The wet cover must be replaced immediately. (TNA 512; LTCA 430)

14. **C**   Pins are not used to secure the aquathermia pad in place. It is a piece of electrical equipment with distilled water flowing through it. Since the distilled water is not in direct contact with the skin, it is a dry heat application. The risk of electrical shock occurs if the unit is punctured. Electrical safety precautions must be practiced. The aquathermia pad is a dry heat application. The temperature of the aquathermia pad is usually set at 105° F. (TNA 519; LTCA 438)

15. **C**   Cold causes the blood vessels to constrict. Less blood, oxygen, and nutrients are carried to the area. Cold applications reduce pain, swelling, circulation, and cool the body. Cold should

be applied immediately after an injury. (TNA 522; LTCA 440)

16. **A** Ice cubes are too bulky in an ice bag. Crushed ice or ice chips allows the bag to conform to the body part and results in more even cooling. The bag should be filled one-half to two-thirds full. Then the excess air is removed. A flannel cover on the bag protects the skin. (TNA 523; LTCA 440)

17. **C** Infections are not usually a complication of local cold applications. Pain, cyanosis, burns, and blisters are possible complications of local cold applications. (TNA 522; LTCA 440)

18. **A** An ice bag is a dry cold application. The cold compress, cold soak, and cool bath are considered moist cold applications. (TNA 522; LTCA 440)

19. **D** The cool water bath is used to reduce body temperature when there is a high fever. (TNA 526; LTCA 440)

20. **A** Vital signs are taken before giving a cool sponge bath. Ice bags are applied to the forehead, axillae, and groin areas (not the feet) to help lower the body temperature. One bath blanket is used to provide the resident with privacy during the bath. (TNA 526–527; LTCA 444–445)

Oxygen Therapy
(p. 78)

1. **C** A nasal cannula is a double-pronged device placed in the nostrils. It is the simplest and most commonly used device to administer oxygen. The resident can eat and talk with the cannula in place. Nasal catheters, oxygen tents, and face masks are used less often. (TNA 537; LTCA 454)

2. **A** Fire safety precautions must be adhered to when oxygen is in use. Oxygen is essential for a fire. It can ignite and cause an explosion. Suctioning and isolation techniques may or may not be used, depending on the resident's condition and diagnosis. Medical asepsis is always important, but is not the most important concern when using oxygen. (TNA 536–537; LTCA 453–455)

3. **C** Nursing assistants never remove the oxygen administration device. Oral hygiene should be given as directed by the nurse. There should be no kinks in the tubing. Safety measures related to fire and the use of oxygen must be followed. (TNA 536–537; LTCA 453–455)

4. **B** Oral hygiene is very important because the resident receiving oxygen often breathes through the mouth. Nursing assistants never turn off the oxygen or adjust the flow rate of the oxygen. The nurse or physician decides if the mask can be changed to a nasal cannula. (TNA 536–537; LTCA 453–455)

5. **C** Oxygen is a colorless gas. It is considered a drug. Oxygen is tasteless and odorless. (TNA 536–537; LTCA 453–455)

Coughing, Deep Breathing Exercises, and Collecting Sputum Specimens
(pp. 78–79)

1. **D** Sputum specimens consist of secretions from the lungs, trachea, and bronchi. Saliva is a thin, clear liquid produced by the salivary glands in the mouth. Secretions from the stomach or a surgical wound would be used to assess those areas. (TNA 538–539; LTCA 455–458)

2. **D** Rinsing the mouth with plain water decreases the amount of saliva and removes any food particles. To void is to urinate. The person should be allowed to use the bathroom, bedpan, or commode chair if he or she needs to void. This will not affect the sputum specimen in any way. Encouraging the resident to cough after two or three deep breaths will help him or her cough up the sputum. Rinsing the mouth with mouthwash or brushing with toothpaste may destroy some microorganisms. (TNA 538–539; LTCA 455–458)

3. **D** Since sputum is examined for microorganisms, blood, or cells, a fresh specimen container is used. This eliminates the need to transfer the specimen and possibly contaminating it. (TNA 538–539; LTCA 455–458)

4. **D** Semi-Fowler's is usually the most comfortable position for coughing and deep breathing. (TNA 538–539; LTCA 455–458)

5. **D** Coughing removes mucus from the respiratory passages. Deep breathing moves air into the lung. Both measures help prevent respiratory complications. The exercises do not prevent bleeding, pain, or cyanosis. (TNA 538–539; LTCA 455–458)

Binders, Support Bandages, and Stockings
(p. 79)

1. **D** Binders provide support or hold dressings in place. They do not prevent blood clots or infection. Binders do not decrease circulation or swelling. (TNA 560–563; LTCA 459–462)

2. **B** Elastic stockings exert pressure on the veins, promoting venous blood flow. This helps prevent the development of thrombi (blood clots). They help to prevent swelling by promoting venous blood flow. (TNA 560–563; LTCA 459–462)

3. **A** An embolus is a blood clot that travels through the vascular system until it lodges in a distant vessel. Thrombi and thrombus are terms that describe a blood clot. The term antiembolus

describes something that would prevent an embolus from forming. (TNA 560–563; LTCA 459–462)

4. **B** A loose and wrinkled binder must be reapplied. A wet binder must be replaced with a new binder. Securing the binder with more pins does not help. (TNA 560–563; LTCA 459–462)

5. **D** The stockings come in many sizes. Thigh-high or knee-length stockings are available. The nurse measures the person to determine the correct size. The stockings are removed at least twice each day. They are applied before the person gets out of bed to prevent the venous blood from pooling in the feet. If the person has been out of bed, the legs should be elevated for 20 minutes before the stockings are applied. (TNA 560–563; LTCA 459–462)

Clearing an Obstructed Airway (Heimlich Maneuver) (p. 80)

1. **A** Large pieces of meat are the most common causes of choking. Other items can cause choking, but are not as common. (TNA 696–701; LTCA 543–545)

2. **C** The resident who is choking will clutch at the throat. The victim will not be able to speak or breathe and will appear pale and cyanotic (bluish discoloration). (TNA 696–701; LTCA 543–545)

3. **A** The Heimlich maneuver is not effective on extremely obese individuals. Chest thrusts are used instead. The maneuver can be used on victims who are standing, sitting, or lying down. (TNA 696–701; LTCA 543–545)

4. **D** Quick, upward thrusts should be given. You should stand behind the victim who is standing. Your hands should be wrapped around the victim's waist. Place your fist in the middle of the abdomen above the navel and below the sternum in order to push on the diaphragm. (TNA 696–701; LTCA 543–545)

5. **C** Properly fitting dentures are not a cause of choking in the elderly. Weakness, chronic illnesses, and poor swallowing reflexes can lead to choking in the elderly. (TNA 696–701; LTCA 543–545)

PART THREE The Skills Evaluation

Section I Preparing for the Skills Evaluation

In addition to the written evaluation, OBRA requires an evaluation of your manual skills. The purpose of the evaluation is to make sure you can correctly perform certain skills. This helps to insure that the person will receive safe and appropriate care. While you learned many skills during your training program, only selected skills are part of the manual evaluation. The National Council of State Boards of Nursing, Inc. has identified essential skills for nursing assistants. Those skills are included in this review book. However, this book is not a textbook or a substitute for proper instruction. Previous nursing assistant education and supervised on-the-job training are also necessary.

During the evaluation, a registered nurse evaluates your performance of certain skills. Being watched by someone as you work is not a new experience. Your instructor evaluated your performance during your nursing assistant course. While you are working, your supervisor evaluates your skills. However, you may be anxious and nervous about the skills examination. The following information can help you prepare for the exam.

1. You were expected to safely and properly perform nursing skills during your nursing assistant course to pass the course. Since you passed the course, you know how to safely and properly perform the necessary nursing skills.
2. These skills are performed daily as part of your nursing care. You receive supervision and on-the-job training from your supervisors. This means that you safely and properly perform these skills every day.
3. The skills evaluated on the manual skills exam are included in this book. These step-by-step checklists can be used to review the skills as often as necessary to prepare for the skills evaluation. You can refer to *Mosby's Textbook for Nursing Assistants* or *Mosby's Textbook for*
Long-Term Care Assistants if you need more information.
4. Practice each skill to increase your confidence. You can practice with another nursing assistant. The nurses, your supervisor, or the inservice director are other resources. Ask the person helping you to use the step-by-step skills guide in this book or those in *Mosby's Textbook for Nursing Assistants* or *Mosby's Textbook for Long-Term Care Assistants*.

Each state has its own policies and procedures for the skills evaluation. However, the following information will provide you with a general overview of what to expect.

1. Testing may be done at community colleges, vocational schools, high school vocational or career centers, long-term care facilities, or hospitals.
2. Some states allow you to choose the location for your manual evaluation. Other states assign you to a specific testing site.
3. In a school or college, the testing area will be a nursing laboratory. Actual resident rooms or in-service departments may be used in long-term care facilities.
4. The testing area will include the furniture and equipment needed to perform the skills.
5. You will be asked to perform randomly selected skills. The skills tested and the number evaluated may vary somewhat from state to state. For example, you may have to perform 5 skills from a list of 25.
6. You are told which skills you are to perform at the time of your evaluation. You do **not** select the skills.
7. You will be given a certain amount of time to perform the required skills.
8. Mannequins and people will be used as "residents," depending on the skills you are to perform.

9. Do not panic if you make a mistake. Tell the evaluator what you did wrong. Then perform the action correctly.

10. Be certain to take whatever equipment you normally take or use at work. Wear a wristwatch with a second hand. You will need it to measure vital signs and to check how much time you have left.

Evaluators will assess other things besides correct skill performance. They will observe for safety practices. How you treat the person and protect resident's rights will also be assessed. Adhering to the following rules will not only help you with the skills examination (even if you are performing the skill on a mannequin), but with your day-to-day care.

1. Identify the person to make certain you are giving care to the right person. Check the identification bracelet with the treatment card or assignment sheet. Also call the person by name.

2. Provide privacy. This involves pulling the privacy curtain around the bed, closing doors, asking visitors to leave the room, and/or moving appropriate screening devices.

3. Always follow the rules of medical asepsis.

4. Make sure the signal light is within the person's reach. Attaching it to the bed or side rail does not mean it can be reached by the person.

5. Make sure the side rails are up, if appropriate. The side rail on the opposite side you are working on should be up. Determine if both side rails should be raised when you are done giving care or when you leave the bedside. They may be considered a restraint if the person does not require them for a specific reason.

6. Use good body mechanics. Raise the bed and overbed table to a good working height.

7. Place the bed in the lowest horizontal position when the person must get out of bed or when you are done giving care.

8. Treat the person with respect. Call the person by the name that he or she prefers. Greet the person in a pleasant and friendly manner. Always explain to the person what you are going to do before beginning the procedure. Also explain what you are doing during the procedure.

9. Communicate with the person while giving care. Focus on the person's needs and interests. Do not talk about yourself or your personal problems.

PART THREE The Skills Evaluation

Section II Skills Competency Review

Universal precautions, body mechanics, communication with the person, and resident's rights are assessed as part of the other manual skills. The guidelines have been included for these skills instead of separate checklists. You will want to adhere to these guidelines as you provide your care.

Universal Precautions (TNA 193; LTCA 143)

- Gloves are worn when touching blood, body fluids, body substances, and mucous membranes. This includes vaginal secretions and semen.
- Gloves are worn for contact with surfaces or items soiled with blood, body fluids, or body substances.
- Gloves are worn when there are cuts, breaks, or openings in the skin.
- Gloves are worn when there is possible contact with mucous membranes, urine, feces, vomitus, dressings, wound drainage, soiled linen, or soiled clothing.
- Gloves are changed after contact with each person.
- Gloves are not washed for reuse.
- Masks, goggles, or face shields are worn when splattering or splashing of blood or body fluids is possible. (This protects your eyes and the mucous membranes of your mouth.)
- Gowns or aprons are worn when splashing, splattering, smearing, or soiling from blood or body fluids is possible.
- Hands and other body parts must be washed immediately if contaminated with blood or body fluids.
- Hands are washed immediately after removing gloves.
- Hands are washed after contact with the person.
- Avoid nicks or cuts when shaving residents.
- Handle razor blades and other sharp objects carefully to avoid injuring the person or yourself.
- Use resuscitation devices when mouth-to-mouth resuscitation is indicated.
- Avoid patient/resident contact when you have open skin wounds or lesions. Discuss the situation with your supervisor.
- Place linen soiled with blood, body fluids, or body substances in leakage-resistant bags.
- Garbage contaminated with blood or body fluids is placed in a biohazard bag.
- Equipment contaminated with blood or body fluids are properly disinfected or disposed of according to facility policy.
- Follow facility policy for the disposal of infective wastes.

- Blood spills are promptly cleaned with a solution of sodium hypochlorite diluted 1:10 with water.

Body Mechanics (TNA 213 ; LTCA 159)

- Stand in good alignment and with a wide base of support.
- Face the direction of the item to be picked up.
- Use the stronger and larger muscles of your body. They are in the shoulders, upper arms, thighs, and hips.
- Keep objects close to your body when you lift, move, or carry them.
- Avoid unnecessary bending and reaching. If possible, have the height of the bed and overbed table level with your waist when you give care. Adjust the bed and table to the proper height.
- To prevent unnecessary twisting, face the area in which you are working.
- Push, slide, or pull heavy objects whenever possible rather than lift them.
- Use both hands and arms when you lift, move, or carry heavy objects.
- Turn your whole body when you change the direction of your movement.
- Work with smooth and even movements. Avoid sudden or jerky motions.
- Get help from a co-worker to move heavy objects or persons.
- Squat to lift heavy objects from the floor and to return them. Push against the strong hip and thigh muscles to raise yourself to a standing position.

Communicating with the Person (TNA 81-83; LTCA 55)

- Understand and respect the individual as a person.
- Call the person by the name that he or she prefers.
- View the person as more than a disease or an illness. The person is a physical, psychological, social, and spiritual human being.
- Appreciate the problems and frustrations the person is experiencing as a result of being sick.
- Recognize and respect the person's rights.
- Explain procedures prior to beginning care.
- Respect the person's religion and culture.
- Use words that mean the same to the person and you.
- Speak in short sentences.
- Avoid using medical terminology and unfamiliar words.
- Avoid using slang or vulgar words.
- Control the loudness and tone of your voice.
- Speak clearly, slowly, and distinctly.
- Communicate in a logical and orderly manner.
- Be specific and factual when presenting information.
- Be brief and concise.
- Ask one question at a time and wait for the answer; do not ask several questions at once.
- Give the person time to process (understand) the information you give.
- Ask questions to be sure you have been understood. Repeat information as often as necessary. Repeat exactly what you said so the person does not have to process a new message. This is especially important for persons with hearing problems.
- Be patient. The person with memory problems may ask the same question several times a day. Do not remind them that you are repeating information. Accept their memory loss as you would any other disability.

Resident Rights (TNA 140-143; LTCA 8 -10)

- Residents of long-term care facilities have certain rights under federal and state laws.
- Residents have rights as citizens of the United States.
- *Right to information*
  - This includes access to all records relating to the resident.

- The resident or legal representative has the right to be fully informed of the person's total health condition in language the person can understand.
- The resident and legal representative have the right to know the resident's doctor, including name, specialty, and how he or she can be contacted.

NOTE: Any request for information should be given to the nurse.

- *Right to refuse treatment*
  - The facility must find out what the resident is refusing and why.

  NOTE: Any refusal of treatment should be reported to the nurse.
- *Privacy and confidentiality*
  - Personal privacy
    - The resident's body must not be exposed unnecessarily.
    - The right to visit with others in private.
    - The right to have telephone conversations in private.
    - The right to send and receive mail without interference by others.
    - Confidentiality is maintained about the resident's care, treatment, medical condition, and medical and financial records.
- *Personal choice*
  - Residents are free to choose their own doctors.
  - They have the right to participate in planning their own care and treatment.
  - This helps with the person's quality of life, dignity, and self-respect.
- *Disputes and grievances*
  - Residents have the right to voice concerns, questions, or complaints about treatment or care without punishment in any way.
  - The facility must promptly try to correct the situation.
- *Work*
  - The resident does not work to receive care, items, or other things or privileges.
  - If the resident desires or needs to work for rehabilitation or activity purposes, it should be part of the resident's care plan.
- *Participation in resident and family groups*
  - Residents have the right to form groups.
  - A resident's family has the right to meet with families of other residents.
  - Residents have the right to take part in social, religious, and community activities.
  - Residents have the right to assistance in getting to and from activities of their choice.
- *Care and security of personal possessions*
  - Residents have the right to keep and use personal items.
  - A person's property must be treated with care and respect.
  - The facility must take reasonable measures to protect the person's property.
    - Items are labeled with the resident's name.
    - The facility must investigate reports of lost, stolen, or damaged items.
- *Freedom from abuse, mistreatment, and neglect*
  - Residents have the right to be free from verbal, sexual, physical, or mental abuse.
  - Residents have the right to be free from involuntary seclusion.
    - Involuntary seclusion is separating the resident from others against his or her will. It can also mean keeping the person confined to a certain area or away from his or her room without consent.
  - No one can abuse, neglect, or mistreat the resident.
  - Nursing facilities must have policies and procedures for investigating suspected or reported cases of resident abuse.
  - Nursing facilities cannot employ persons who have been convicted of abusing, neglecting, or mistreating other individuals.

- *Freedom from restraints*
  - Residents have the right not to have body movements restricted.
  - A doctor's order is necessary for restraints.
  - Restraints cannot be used for the convenience of the staff or to discipline a resident.
- *Quality of life*
  - Nursing facilities must care for residents in a manner that promotes dignity, self-worth, and physical, psychological, and emotional well-being.
  - The resident is spoken to in a polite and courteous manner.
  - The resident is provided good, honest, and thoughtful care.
  - Activities are important for a resident's quality of life.
    - Nursing facilities must provide activity programs that meet the interests and physical, mental, and psychosocial needs of each resident.
  - The environment of the facility must promote quality of life.
    - The facility must be clean, safe, and as home-like as possible.

SKILL 1
Handwashing (TNA 188; LTCA 139)

STEPS	S	U	COMMENTS
1. Gathered equipment.			
2. Pushed watch up 4 to 5 inches.			
3. Stood away from sink; did not allow clothes to touch the sink.			
4. Turned faucet on, using a paper towel if facility policy.			
5. Adjusted water so that it felt warm and comfortable.			
6. Tossed paper towel used to turn on faucet into the wastebasket.			
7. Wet wrists and hands thoroughly under running water keeping hands lower than elbows.			
8. Applied soap or detergent to hands. a. Rinsed bar soap before use.			
9. Rubbed palms together to work up good lather.			

10. Washed each hand and wrist thoroughly for 1–2 minutes.
   a. Washed between fingers.
   b. Rubbed fingertips into palms in circular motion.			

11. Returned soap to soap dish, if bar soap used.			
12. Rinsed hands thoroughly from wrists to fingertips keeping hands down.			
13. Dried hands and wrists with paper towels by patting dry.			
14. Discarded wet paper towels in wastebasket.			
15. Turned off faucet with clean dry paper towel and discarded in wastebasket.			

SKILL 2
Applying a Jacket or Vest Restraint (TNA 171; LTCA 124)

STEPS	S	U	COMMENTS
1. Obtained a jacket or vest restraint in the correct size.			
2. Found assistance if needed.			
3. Washed hands.			

4. Identified resident:
   a. Checked ID bracelet.
   b. Called resident by name.			

5. Explained procedure to resident.			
6. Provided for privacy.			
7. Assisted the resident to a sitting position by locking arms with the resident.			
8. Slipped the resident's arm through the arm holes of the restraint with the free hand, and applied the restraint according to manufacturer's instructions.			
9. Made sure there were no wrinkles in the front or back of the restraint.			
10. Helped the resident to lie or sit down.			
11. Brought the ties through the slots.			
12. Made sure the resident was comfortable and in good body alignment.			
13. Tied the straps to the bed frame, bed springs, or under chair. Used a quick-release knot or a facility-approved knot.			
14. Made sure the knot was not too tight. Able to slide flat hand between the restraint and the resident. Adjusted straps if necessary.			
15. Placed the signal light within reach.			
16. Raised the side rails and made sure they were padded.			
17. Unscreened the resident.			
18. Washed hands.			
19. Checked the restraint every 15 minutes.			

20. Removed the restraint every 2 hours and repositioned the resident.
   a. Met the resident's needs for food, fluids, and elimination.
   b. Gave skin care and performed range-of-motion exercises.
   c. Reapplied restraint.			

21. Reported observations to the nurse.			

SKILL 3			
Moving and Turning a Resident in Bed (TNA 230; LTCA 171)			
STEPS	S	U	COMMENTS
1. Washed hands.			

2. Identified resident:
   a. Checked ID bracelet.
   b. Called resident by name.			

3. Explained procedure to the resident.			
4. Provided privacy.			
5. Locked bed wheels.			
6. Raised the bed.			
7. Lowered head of the bed to a level appropriate for the resident.			
8. Went to side of bed opposite of which resident will be turned. a. Opposite rail up.			
9. Lowered closest side rail.			

10. Moved resident to closest side of bed.
   a. Stood so that feet were 12 inches apart and one foot was in front of the other. Flexed knees.
   b. Crossed resident's arms over chest.
   c. Placed arm under resident's neck and shoulders, grasping far shoulder.
   d. Placed other arm under resident's midback.
   e. Moved upper part of the resident's body toward self.
   f. Put one arm under the resident's waist and other under the thighs.
   g. Moved lower part of resident's body toward self by rocking backward.
   h. Repeated for legs and feet. Arms were placed under resident's thighs and calves.			

11. Crossed resident's arms over chest and nearest leg over the other leg.			
12. Raised side rails and went to other side. a. Lowered that side rail.			

13. Stood so that feet were 12 inches apart.
   a. Flexed knees.
   b. Kept back straight.			

14. Put one hand on the resident's shoulder. a. Other hand on far hip.			
15. Rolled the resident toward self gently.			

16. Positioned resident for comfort and good body alignment.
   a. Positioned pillow behind back for support.
   b. Put a pillow under head and shoulder.
   c. Placed a pillow in front of the bottom leg.
   d. Placed top leg on pillow in a flexed position.
   e. Supported arm and hand on a small pillow.			

17. Placed signal light within resident's reach.			

STEPS	S	U	COMMENTS
18. Raised the side rail.			
19. Lowered bed to lowest horizontal position.			
20. Unscreened (pulled back drapes) the resident.			
21. Washed hands.			

SKILL 4
Applying a Transfer (Gait) Belt (TNA 236; LTCA 176)

STEPS	S	U	COMMENTS
1. Washed hands.			

2. Identified resident:
    a. Checked ID bracelet.
    b. Called resident by name.			

3. Explained procedure to the resident.			
4. Provided privacy.			
5. Assisted resident to a sitting position.			
6. Applied belt around resident's waist over clothing.			
7. Tightened belt till snug. a. Does not cause discomfort or impair breathing.			
8. Made sure a woman's breasts were not caught under the belt.			
9. Placed buckle off center in front or in back for resident's comfort.			
10. Prepared to transfer or ambulate.			

SKILL 5 **Transferring the Resident to a Chair or Wheelchair** (TNA 238–240; LTCA 177–179)			
STEPS	S	U	COMMENTS
1. Explained procedure to resident.			

2. Collected necessary equipment:
  a. Wheelchair or armchair.
  b. One or two bath blankets or lap robe.
  c. Clothing or robe and shoes.
  d. Paper or sheet for the bottom linen.
  e. Transfer (gait) belt if needed.
  f. Special cushion if used.			

3. Washed hands.			

4. Identified resident.
  a. Checked ID bracelet.
  b. Called person by name.			

5. Provided for privacy.			
6. Decided which side of bed to use based on person's strongest side. a. Moved furniture to provide space.			
7. Placed chair or wheelchair at head of bed. a. Back of the chair or wheelchair was even with the headboard.			

8. Placed folded bath blanket or cushion in seat.
  a. Locked wheelchair wheels.
  b. Raised the footrests.			

9. Made sure bed in lowest position. a. Made sure bed wheels locked.			
10. Fan-folded linens to foot of bed.			
11. Helped resident put on clothing or robe.			
12. Placed paper or sheet under resident's feet protecting bottom sheet. a. Put shoes on resident.			
13. Helped resident dangle. a. Made sure resident's feet touched floor.			
14. Applied transfer belt.			

15. Helped resident to stand. If transfer belt was used:
  a. Stood in front of resident.
  b. Had resident put fists on bed by thighs.
  c. Made sure resident's feet were flat on floor.
  d. Had resident lean forward.
  e. Grasped transfer belt at each side.
  f. Braced knees against resident's knees.
  g. Blocked resident's feet with own feet.
  h. Asked resident to push fists into bed and to stand on count of "3."
  i. Pulled resident into standing position while straightening own knees.			

STEPS	S	U	COMMENTS

16. If transfer belt not used:
   a. Stood in front of resident.
   b. Had resident place fists on bed by thighs.
   c. Made sure resident's feet were flat on floor.
   d. Placed hands under resident's arms with hands around the shoulder blades.
   e. Had resident lean forward.
   f. Braced knees against resident's knees and blocked resident's feet with own feet.
   g. Asked resident to push fists into bed and to stand on count of "3."
   h. Pulled resident into standing position while straightened own knees.			

17. Supported resident into standing position.
   a. Held transfer belt or resident's shoulder blades.
   b. Continued to block resident's feet and knees with own feet and knees.			

18. Turned resident until able to grasp far arm of chair.
   a. Legs touched edge of chair.
   b. Turned resident until other armrest was grasped.			

19. Lowered resident into chair while bending own hips and knees. a. Resident assisted by leaning forward and bending elbows and knees.			
20. Made sure buttocks were at back of chair. a. Positioned resident in good alignment.			
21. Positioned feet on footrests.			
22. Covered resident's lap and legs with lap robe or bath blanket. a. Did not allow lap robe or blanket to touch floor or wheels.			
23. Removed transfer belt.			
24. Positioned chair as resident preferred.			
25. Placed signal light and other necessary items within reach. a. Straightened the unit.			
26. Unscreened the resident.			
27. Washed hands.			

28. Reported to nurse:
   a. Pulse (if taken).
   b. How activity was tolerated.
   c. Any resident complaints.
   d. Amount of assistance needed to transfer resident.			

29. Reversed procedure to return resident to bed.			

SKILL 6 Repositioning a Resident in a Wheelchair			
STEPS	**S**	**U**	**COMMENTS**
1. Explained procedure.			
2. Provided privacy.			
3. Locked wheels of wheelchair			
4. Raised footrests.			
5. Asked resident to fold arms in front of chest. a. Crossed resident's arms, if unable to do so.			
6. Stood behind resident.			
7. Bent down toward resident with hips and knees.			
8. Slid arms under resident's upper arms and grasped resident's wrists.			
9. Asked resident to push with feet on count of "3."			
10. Pulled resident to back of chair on count of "3."			
11. Made sure the resident's back and buttocks are against back of chair.			
12. Made sure feet are on wheelchair footrests.			
13. If paralyzed, positioned arm on pillow with wrist at a slight upward angle.			
14. Covered resident with lap blanket if one used. a. Made sure blanket did not dangle on floor or wheels.			

SKILL 7			
Making an Unoccupied (Open) Bed (TNA 269–274; LTCA 214–218)			
STEPS	**S**	**U**	**COMMENTS**
1. Washed hands.			
2. Took linen to bedside and placed over back of chair at bedside.			
3. Elevated bed to working height and locked wheels.			
4. Pushed mattress to top of bed.			
5. Placed mattress pad on bed (even with head and foot ends of mattress).			
6. Placed bottom sheet lengthwise in center of bed and unfolded, tucked in and mitered corners if using flat sheets.			
7. Placed drawsheet and tucked in.			
8. Placed folded top sheet in center of bed with wide hem at top of mattress, and unfolded with wrong side up. a. Tucked sheet in and mitered corners.			
9. Placed bedspread smooth side up in center of bed, unfolded and tucked in securely and mitered corners. a. Repeated steps 6 through 9.			
10. Made cuff at top of bed with top linens.			
11. Put pillow slip on by pulling pillow into it.			
12. Placed pillow at head of bed. a. Open end away from door.			
13. Returned bed to lowest position.			
14. Washed hands.			

SKILL 8
Making an Occupied Bed (TNA 274–275; LTCA 219–220)

STEPS	S	U	COMMENTS
1. Identified resident: a. Checked ID bracelet. b. Called resident by name.			
2. Explained procedure to the resident.			
3. Took linen to bedside and placed over back of chair in order of use.			
4. Washed hands.			
5. Provided for privacy.			
6. Raised bed to working height.			
7. Checked side rails and raised, if necessary.			
8. Applied gloves.			
9. Loosened top linens at foot of bed. a. Removed pillow (unless resident might be uncomfortable). b. Placed pillow on chair.			
10. Removed bedspread a. Folded toward foot of bed approximately in half, then quarter fold. b. Removed from bed. c. Placed over back of a chair.			
11. Placed bath blanket over top sheet.			
12. Removed top sheet from beneath bath blanket. a. Placed in soiled linen hamper or in an appropriate location.			
13. Checked side rail up on opposite side of bed, raised if necessary.			
14. Lowered side rail on same side and assisted resident to turn onto side.			
15. Loosened drawsheet and bottom sheet.			
16. Fan-folded drawsheet to center of bed (toward resident's back).			
17. Fan-folded soiled bottom sheet to center of bed.			
18. Placed lengthwise folded flat sheet smoothly on bed with narrow hem at foot of bed even with food of mattress, or placed fitted bottom sheet lengthwise on bed.			
19. Fan-folded clean bottom sheet to center of bed next to soiled bottom sheet.			
20. Tucked near half of bottom sheet under mattress at head of bed. a. Mitered corner.			
21. Placed clean drawsheet on bed.			
22. Tucked both sheets in.			
23. Placed liftsheet if indicated. a. Located on bed under shoulder to knees.			
24. Assisted resident in turning to clean side of bed.			

STEPS	S	U	COMMENTS
25. Raised side rails.			
26. Went to opposite side of bed and lowered side rails.			
27. Loosened linens.			
28. Removed soiled bottom sheet and drawsheet. 　a. Rolled them together into bundle.			
29. Unfolded bottom sheet and tucked under mattress at head of bed. 　a. Mitered corner.			
30. Unfolded drawsheet.			
31. Tightened bottom sheet and drawsheet. 　a. Tucked under mattress.			
32. Unfolded liftsheet and smoothed, if used.			
33. Assisted resident to center of bed.			
34. Changed pillowslip. 　a. Placed pillow under resident's head. 　b. Open end away from door. 　c. Placed seam toward head of bed.			
35. Placed wide seam of clean top sheet, wrong side up, over bath blanket.			
36. Opened sheet by unfolding toward foot of bed.			
37. Removed bath blanket from under top sheet. 　a. Placed with other soiled linen or in hamper.			
38. Placed bedspread over sheet.			
39. Tucked in bottom of top bedding. 　a. Mitered corners.			
40. Placed bed in lowest position.			
41. Raised or lowered side rails, as appropriate.			
42. Ensured resident's comfort.			
43. Placed signal light within reach.			
44. Placed soiled linen in linen hamper.			
45. Removed gloves.			
46. Washed hands.			

SKILL 9
Brushing the Resident's Teeth (TNA 287; LTCA 233)

STEPS	S	U	COMMENTS
1. Washed hands.			
2. Gathered equipment and arranged on table.			

3. Identified resident.
  a. Checked ID bracelet.
  b. Called person by name.			

4. Explained procedure.			
5. Provided for privacy.			
6. Raised head of resident's bed.			
7. Lowered side rail and placed over-the-bed table in front of the resident.			
8. Applied gloves.			
9. Placed towel over resident's chest.			

10. Allowed resident to brush teeth (assist as needed).
  a. Brushed teeth back and forth.
  b. Positioned brush at 45° angle against inside of front teeth and brushed from crown to gum with short strokes.
  c. Held brush horizontally against inner surfaces of teeth and brushed back and forth.
  d. Positioned brush on biting surfaces of teeth and brushed back and forth.			

11. Flossed resident's teeth by stretching 18 inches of floss between middle fingers of each hand and moving floss gently up and down between teeth. a. Moved to new section of floss after every second tooth.			
12. Had resident rinse mouth with mouthwash.			
13. Held emesis basin under chin to collect expectoration.			
14. Unscreened resident.			
15. Cleaned equipment.			
16. Removed gloves.			
17. Washed hands.			

18. Reported and recorded observations
  a. Dry, cracked, swollen, blistered lips.
  b. Redness, swelling, irritation, sores, or white patches.
  c. Bleeding, swelling, excessive redness of gums.			

SKILL 10
Giving a Partial Bath (TNA 301; LTCA 247)

STEPS	S	U	COMMENTS
1. Identified resident. a. Checked ID bracelet. b. Called person by name.			
2. Explained procedure.			
3. Offered bedpan or urinal. a. Provided privacy.			
4. Washed hands.			
5. Collected linen for a closed bed. Placed linen on chair.			
6. Collected equipment: a. Wash basin. b. Soap dish with soap. c. Bath thermometer. d. Washcloth. e. Two bath towels and two face towels. f. Bath blanket. g. Gown or pajamas. h. Oral hygiene equipment. i. Body lotion and talcum powder. j. Deodorant or antiperspirant. k. Brush and comb. l. Other toiletries requested by resident. m. Paper towels.			
7. Arranged equipment on over-the-bed table. a. Placed supplies to be used later on the bedside stand.			
8. Closed doors and windows to prevent drafts.			
9. Removed top linen. a. Covered resident with bath blanket.			
10. Placed paper towels on over-the-bed table.			
11. Filled wash basin with water 110°F to 115°F (43° to 46°C).			
12. Placed basin on over-the-bed table on top of paper towels.			
13. Lowered near side rail.			
14. Washed resident's face. a. Placed a towel over chest. b. Made a mitt with a washcloth. c. Washed eyes with water only. Inner aspect to outer. Farthest eye first. Repeated with near eye. d. Asked resident if soap is used on face. e. Washed face, ears, and neck. Rinsed and dried well. Used towel on resident's chest.			
15. Helped resident move to closest side of bed.			
16. Removed gown. a. Did not expose resident.			
17. Placed bath towel lengthwise under far arm.			

STEPS	S	U	COMMENTS
18. Supported arm with palm of hand under resident's elbow. a. Resident's forearm should rest on forearm.			
19. Washed arm, shoulder, and underarm with long, firm strokes. Rinsed and patted dry.			

20. Placed wash basin on towel.
    a. Put resident's hand into water.
    b. Washed hand well.
    c. Cleaned under fingernails with an orange stick or nail file.			

21. Removed wash basin and dried hand well. a. Covered arm with bath blanket.			
22. Repeated steps 17 through 21 for near arm.			
23. Turned resident onto far side. a. Kept properly covered with bath blanket.			

24. Uncovered back and buttocks.
    a. Did not expose resident.
    b. Placed towel lengthwise on bed along back.			

25. Washed back working from neck to buttocks.
    a. Used long, firm continuous strokes.
    b. Rinsed and dried well.			

26. Changed water for perineal care.			

27. Let resident wash perineum.
    a. Adjusted over-the-bed table so resident could reach.
    b. Placed signal light within reach.
    c. Asked person to signal when through.
    d. Made sure resident understood what was to be done.
    e. Answered signal light promptly.
    f. Provided perineal care if resident could not.			

28. Applied deodorant or antiperspirant if requested.			
29. Helped resident put on a clean gown or pajamas.			
30. Assisted with hair care.			
31. Made bed. a. Lowered bed to lowest horizontal position.			

32. Made sure resident was comfortable.
    a. Signal light within reach.
    b. Made sure side rails were up if needed.			

33. Emptied and cleaned wash basin. a. Returned equipment.			
34. Wiped off over-the-bed table with paper towels. a. Discarded paper towels.			
35. Unscreened resident.			
36. Placed soiled linen in hamper.			
37. Washed hands.			

SKILL 11 Giving Perineal Care (TNA 309–311; LTCA 256–259)			
STEPS	S	U	COMMENTS
1. Washed hands.			
2. Identified resident. a. Checked ID bracelet. b. Called person by name.			
3. Explained procedure.			
4. Collected equipment.			
5. Set up equipment.			
6. Applied gloves.			
7. Provided for privacy.			
8. Raised bed to working level.			
9. Lowered side rail on the side on which you are working.			
10. Covered resident with bath blanket.			
11. Moved top linens to the foot of the bed.			
12. Placed waterproof pad under buttocks.			
13. Offer bedpan or urinal.			
14. Draped the bath blanket with one corner between the resident's legs. a. Wrapped blanket around each leg.			
15. Raised side rail.			
16. Filled the wash basin with water (105°–110° F).			
17. Wet washcloths (or cotton balls) in the basin.			
18. Lowered side rail.			
19. Helped resident flex knees and spread legs.			
20. Folded bath blanket back.			

21. Washed perineal area.
 a. Females:
  1) Separated labia.
  2) Using downward strokes, cleaned front to back.
  3) Repeated using additional cloths or cotton balls.
 b. Males:
  1) Grasped the penis.
  2) Cleaned tip of penis using circular motion.
  3) Retracted foreskin if resident was not circumcised.			

22. Rinsed the perineal area using the same procedure used to wash.			
23. Turned the resident onto side. a. Cleaned the anal area by washing front to back.			
24. Patted perineal area and anal area dry.			
25. Removed waterproof pad.			

STEPS	S	U	COMMENTS

26. Removed bath blanket.
   a. Repositioned the resident.
   b. Applied top linens.			

27. Raised side rail and lowered bed.			
28. Emptied and cleaned equipment.			
29. Removed gloves.			
30. Washed hands.			

SKILL 12
Catheter Care (TNA 355; LTCA 296)

STEPS	S	U	COMMENTS
1. Washed hands.			

2. Identified resident.
  a. Checked ID bracelet.
  b. Called person by name.			

3. Explained procedure.			
4. Gathered equipment.			
5. Provided for privacy.			
6. Applied gloves.			
7. Raised bed to working level.			
8. Lowered side rail.			
9. Placed bed protector under resident.			
10. Covered resident with bath blanket.			
11. Performed peri-care.			
12. Had resident lie on back and flex knees.			
13. Exposed genitalia.			
14. Opened catheter care kit and applied antiseptic to applicators if available. a. Wet washcloth and applied soap.			
15. Females: Separated labia. Males: Retracted foreskin of uncircumcised male.			
16. Applied antiseptic solution with applicators to the head of penis or to area inside labia. a. Washed head of penis or area inside labia with washcloth.			
17. Discarded applicator after one stroke. a. Rotated washcloth mitt to expose a clean area after one stroke.			
18. Cleaned catheter with antiseptic solution on cotton ball, or with washcloth, from meatus down catheter approximately 4 inches.			
19. Taped catheter properly to thigh.			
20. Removed bed protector.			
21. Removed bath blanket and returned top linens to proper position.			
22. Raised side rails.			
23. Lowered bed to lowest position.			
24. Unscreened resident.			
25. Cleaned and returned equipment to proper place.			
26. Removed gloves.			
27. Washed hands.			
29. Reported observations.			

SKILL 13 **Positioning Urinary Tubing** (TNA 354; LTCA 295)			
STEPS	**S**	**U**	**COMMENTS**
1. Washed your hands.			

2. Identified resident.
   a. Checked ID bracelet.
   b. Called person by name.			

3. Explained procedure to resident.			
4. Provided for privacy.			
5. Lowered side rail on the side of the urinary drainage bag.			
6. Folded back linens to expose the urinary tubing.			
7. Make sure drainage bag was attached to bed frame. a. Made sure drainage bag was below the level of resident's bladder.			
8. Taped catheter on: Male: to top of thigh. Female: to inner thigh. a. Made sure enough slack on catheter to prevent pressure at urethra.			
9. Coiled tubing on bed. a. Made sure no kinks in tubing.			

10. Using clip provided or pinned tubing to bottom sheet.
   a. Placed rubber band around tubing with clove hitch.
   b. Passed a safety pin through loops.
   c. Pinned to bottom sheet.			

11. Covered resident.			
12. Made resident comfortable.			
13. Raised side rail.			
14. Placed signal light within reach.			
15. Unscreened resident.			
16. Removed any soiled linen or equipment.			
17. Washed hands.			
18. Reported observations.			

SKILL 14 **Measuring Intake and Output** (TNA 415; LTCA 345)			
STEPS	**S**	**U**	**COMMENTS**
1. Washed hands.			

2. Identified resident.
    a. Checked ID bracelet.
    b. Called person by name.			

3. Explained procedure.			
4. Applied gloves.			

5. Measured intake:
    a. Poured liquid remaining in serving container into graduate.
    b. Measured the amount at eye level.
    c. Checked conversion table for the amount of serving.
    d. Subtracted remaining amount from full serving amount.
    e. Repeated steps for all remaining liquids.
    f. Totaled (added above amounts) for the intake.			

6. Measured output:
    a. Poured liquid into graduate.
    b. Measured at eye level.
    c. Recorded amount and time on I&O record.
    d. Cleaned and returned graduate to its proper place.
    e. Cleaned and returned bedpan or commode container to its
       proper place.			

7. Removed gloves and washed hands.			
8. Reported and recorded observations.			

SKILL 15 Feeding the Resident (TNA 418; LTCA 348)			
STEPS	S	U	COMMENTS
1. Washed hands.			
2. Identified resident. a. Checked ID bracelet. b. Called person by name.			
3. Positioned resident in sitting position.			
4. Brought tray to resident. a. Checked resident's ID bracelet with dietary card.			
5. Placed napkin across resident's chest.			
6. Explained what is on tray.			
7. Served foods in order preferred by resident. a. Alternated between solid and liquid foods.			
8. Use spoon for safety. a. Filled no more than 2/3 full.			
9. Allowed time for chewing and swallowing.			
10. Used a straw for liquids if resident cannot drink out of a glass.			
11. Wiped excess food and liquids off mouth.			
12. Noted amounts and type of foods eaten.			
13. Measured intake.			
14. Provided oral hygiene.			
15. Provided for safety and comfort.			
16. Washed hands.			
17. Reported observations.			

SKILL 16
Measuring the Oral Temperature (TNA 433; LTCA 364)

STEPS	S	U	COMMENTS
1. Washed hands.			

2. Identified resident.
    a. Checked ID bracelet.
    b. Called person by name.			

3. Explained procedure.			
4. Asked if resident had drunk, eaten, smoked, or chewed gum within last 15 minutes.			
5. Applied gloves.			

6. Prepared thermometer.
    a. Rinsed thermometer in cool water if soaking in disinfectant solution.
    b. Shook mercury down below 96° F holding thermometer by handle.			

7. Applied thermometer cover.			
8. Placed bulb of thermometer in resident's mouth under tongue. a. Instructed resident to keep mouth closed.			
9. Left in for 3 minutes.			

10. Removed thermometer.
    a. Held stem.
    b. Removed cover.			

11. Read thermometer.			
12. Recorded temperature.			
13. Returned thermometer to proper container.			
14. Removed gloves.			
15. Washed hands.			

SKILL 17			
Measuring Pulse (TNA 445; LTCA 375)			
STEPS	**S**	**U**	**COMMENTS**
1. Washed hands.			

2. Identified resident.
    a. Checked ID bracelet.
    b. Called person by name.			

3. Explained procedure.			
4. Found resident's radial pulse by placing middle three fingers on palm side of resident's wrist on thumb side, next to the bone. a. Did not use thumb.			
5. Counted the beats for 30 seconds times 2, if regular. a. Counted for 1 minute if irregular.			

6. Recorded the pulse rate.
    a. Noted rhythm.
    b. Noted strength.			

7. Made resident comfortable.			
8. Washed hands.			

9. Reported:
    a. Irregular rate.
    b. Irregular rhythm.
    c. Rates below 60 or above 100 beats per minute.			

SKILL 18
Measuring Respirations (TNA 449; LTCA 378)

STEPS	S	U	COMMENTS
1. Washed hands.			

2. Identified resident.
   a. Checked ID bracelet.
   b. Called person by name.			

3. Explained procedure. Note: Do not tell resident that the respirations are being measured as this will alter rate. Usually taken with the pulse but may need to explain the need for silence.			
4. Observed rise and fall of chest.			
5. Counted respirations for 30 seconds times 2, if regular. a. Counted respirations for 1 minute if irregular.			
6. Recorded respirations.			
7. Noted any irregularity.			
8. Washed hands.			

9. Reported any:
   a. Irregular rate.
   b. Respirations that are shallow, abdominal, or difficult.			

SKILL 19
Measuring Blood Pressure (TNA 302; LTCA 303–305)

STEPS	S	U	COMMENTS

1. Collected equipment:
  a. sphygmomanometer (blood pressure cuff)
  b. stethoscope
  c. alcohol wipes
  d. paper and pen			

2. Washed hands.			
3. Identified resident and explain what you are going to do.			
4. Provided privacy.			
5. Wiped stethoscope earpieces and diaphragm with wipes.			
6. Positioned resident in a sitting or lying position.			
7. Positioned resident's arm level with heart. Palm is up.			
8. Stood no more than 3 feet away from sphygmomanometer. Placed mercury model vertical, on a flat surface, and at eye level. Placed aneroid type directly in front of you.			
9. Exposed upper arm.			
10. Expelled remaining air from cuff. Close valve on bulb.			
11. Located brachial artery at inner aspect of elbow.			
12. Placed arrow mark on cuff over brachial artery. Wrap cuff around arm at least 1 inch above elbow. Cuff must be even and snug.			
13. Placed stethoscope earpieces in your ears.			
14. Located radial artery. Inflated cuff until unable to feel radial pulse. Inflate cuff 30 mm Hg more.			
15. Positioned stethoscope diaphragm over brachial artery.			
16. Deflated cuff 2 to 4 millimeters per second.			
17. Noted point of first sound (systolic reading).			
18. Continued to deflate cuff. Noted point where sound disappears for diastolic reading.			
19. Deflated cuff completely and remove from arm. Removed stethoscope from your ears.			
20. Recorded resident's name and blood pressure on paper.			
21. Returned cuff to case or wall holder.			
22. Made sure resident was comfortable and signal light was within reach. Unscreened resident.			
23. Cleaned stethoscope with wipes and return equipment.			
24. Washed your hands.			
25. Reported blood pressure to nurse. Recorded in proper place.			

SKILL 20 **Performing Range-of-Motion Exercises (The Lower Leg)** (TNA 461–463; LTCA 390)			
STEPS	**S**	**U**	**COMMENTS**
1. Washed hands.			

2. Identified resident.
    a. Checked ID bracelet.
    b. Called person by name.			

3. Explained procedure.			
4. Elevated bed to working height.			
5. Positioned resident in supine position, if allowed. a. Resident kept in good alignment.			
6. Covered resident with bath blanket. a. Fan-folded top linens to foot of bed.			
7. Exposed only body part to be exercised.			
8. Performed each motion 5 to 6 times on each side.			
Knee			
1. Placed one hand under knee and other under the ankle supporting the leg.			
2. Flexion-Extension a. Bent and straightened knee.			
Ankle			
1. Placed one hand under foot and other under ankle supporting the part.			

2. Dorsiflexion-Plantar Flexion
    a. With leg straight, bent foot toward chest.
    b. Bent foot down.			

3. Inversion-Eversion a. Turned foot in and out.			
Foot			

1. Pronation-Supination
    a. Turned outside of foot up and inside down.
    b. Turned inside of foot up and the outside down.			

Toes			
1. Flexion-Extension a. Bent and straightened toes.			
2. Abduction-Adduction a. Spread toes apart.			

STEPS	S	U	COMMENTS
Post procedure			
1. Lowered bed.			
2. Provided for comfort.			
3. Raised or lowered side rails as instructed by nurse.			
4. Washed hands.			

5. Reported
   a. time exercises performed.
   b. joints that were exercised.
   c. number of times exercises were performed on each joint.
   d. any complaints of pain, signs of stiffness, or spasm.
   e. degree to which resident participated in exercises.			

SKILL 21			
Helping the Resident to Stand and Walk (TNA 466–467; LTCA 394–395)			
STEPS	**S**	**U**	**COMMENTS**
1. Washed hands.			
2. Identified resident. a. Checked ID bracelet. b. Called person by name.			
3. Explained procedure.			
4. Gathered equipment.			
5. Provided for privacy.			
6. Put bed in lowest position. a. Locked wheels.			
7. Lowered side rail.			
8. Fan-folded top linens to foot of bed.			
9. Placed slippers or shoes on resident.			
10. Assisted resident to sit on side of bed (dangle). a. Had resident bend knees. b. Rolled resident towards self. c. Placed one arm over knees and grasped legs from behind. d. Placed one arm under far shoulder. e. One a count of "3," used a smooth motion, brought resident's feet over edge of bed (resident's trunk was upright). f. Braced knees against resident's knees for support and placed hand over resident's shoulders.			
11. When resident was steady, applied transfer (gait) belt snugly around waist.			
12. Brought resident to edge of bed.			
13. Brought resident to a standing position. a. Faced resident. b. Asked resident to place hands on shoulders. c. Grasped transfer (gait) belt securely at sides. d. Braced resident's feet and knees with own; own knees were bent. e. Brought resident into a standing position by straightening own knees.			
14. Stood at resident's side and grasped belt in back with an underhand grasp.			
15. Encouraged resident to ambulate normally.			
16. Assisted resident to ambulate distance as tolerated or to destination.			

STEPS	S	U	COMMENTS
Returning resident to bed			
1. Assisted resident to side of bed.			
2. Had resident stand in front of bed. a. Backs of the knees were touching the bed.			
3. Asked resident to place hands on your shoulders.			
4. Grasped sides of transfer (gait) belt.			
5. Lowered resident onto the bed by bending own knees.			
6. Removed transfer (gait) belt.			

7. Assisted resident to lie down.
    a. Stood slightly to side of resident.
    b. Placed your arm behind resident's back and grasped far shoulder.
    c. Bent knees and placed other arm under resident's legs.
    d. With a count of "3," slowly brought resident's legs around and placed on bed.			

8. Removed slippers or shoes.			
9. Positioned resident in good body alignment and provided for comfort.			
10. Placed call light within reach.			
11. Raised side rail.			
12. Washed hands.			

13. Reported observations.
    a. Distance ambulated.
    b. How activity tolerated.			

SKILL 22 **Measuring and Recording Weight and Height** (TNA 498; LTCA 413)			
STEPS	**S**	**U**	**COMMENTS**
Weight			
1. Washed hands.			

2. Identified resident.
    a. Checked ID bracelet.
    b. Called person by name.			

3. Explained procedure.			

4. Asked resident to urinate.
    a. Offered bedpan or urinal if appropriate.
    b. Assisted to bathroom, if necessary.			

5. Provided privacy.			
6. Asked resident to remove shoes or slippers.			
7. Assisted resident onto scale.			
8. Adjusted scale.			
9. Read and recorded measurement.			
Height			
1. Assisted resident to stand erect with back to meter for safety.			
2. Adjusted height meter to top of head.			
3. Noted height in inches or centimeters.			
4. Assisted resident into chair.			
5. Assisted resident with shoes or slippers if appropriate.			
6. Ensured resident comfort.			
7. Recorded measurements.			
8. Washed hands.			

SKILL 23
Applying Knee-Length Elastic Stockings (TNA 560; LTCA 460)

STEPS	S	U	COMMENTS
1. Washed hands.			

2. Identified resident.
   a. Checked ID bracelet.
   b. Called person by name.			

3. Explained procedure.			
4. Obtained elastic stockings in the correct size.			
5. Raised bed for good body mechanics.			
6. Lowered side rail.			
7. Positioned resident in a supine position.			
8. Exposed legs. a. Fan-folded top linens toward resident.			
9. Held foot and heel of stocking. a. Gathered up stocking.			
10. Supported resident's foot at the heel.			
11. Slipped foot of stocking over toes, foot, and heel.			
12. Pulled stocking up over leg so it was even and snug.			
13. Made sure stocking was not twisted. a. No creases or wrinkles.			
14. Repeated steps 9 through 13 for other leg.			
15. Returned top linens to cover resident.			

16. Made sure resident was comfortable.
   a. Raised side rail.
   b. Placed signal light within reach.			

17. Lowered the bed to lowest horizontal position.			
18. Unscreened resident.			
19. Washed hands.			
20. Reported that stockings were applied and time applied.			

SKILL 24			
Clearing the Obstructed Airway (Heimlich Maneuver)—The Conscious Adult (TNA 698; LTCA 544)			
STEPS	S	U	COMMENTS
1. Asked victim if choking.			
2. Checked if victim could cough or speak.			

3. Called for help while performed Heimlich maneuver (abdominal thrusts) on victim standing or sitting.
  a. Stood behind victim.
  b. Wrapped arms around victim's waist.
  c. Made a fist with one hand. Placed thumb side of fist against victim's abdomen. Positioned fist in middle above navel and below end of sternum.
  d. Grasped fist with other hand.
  e. Pressed fist and hand into victim's abdomen with a quick, upward thrust.
  f. Repeated abdominal thrust until object was expelled or victim lost consciousness.			

SKILL 25			
Denture Care (TNA 293–294; LTCA 238–239)			
STEPS	S	U	COMMENTS
1. Washed hands.			

2. Identified resident.
    a. Checked ID bracelet.
    b. Called person by name.			

3. Explained procedure.			
4. Provided privacy.			
5. Lowered side rail if up.			
6. Placed a towel over resident's chest.			
7. Put on gloves.			
8. Asked resident to remove dentures and placed in kidney (emesis) basin.			

9. Removed dentures if resident unable.
Upper denture:
    a. Grasped with thumb and index finger on one hand.
    b. Moved denture up and down slightly to break seal.
    c. Gently removed and placed in kidney basin.
Lower denture:
    a. Grasped with thumb and index finger.
    b. Turned slightly and lifted out of mouth.
    c. Placed in kidney basin.			

10. Raised or lowered side rail as necessary.			
11. Took kidney basin, denture cup, brush, and denture cleaner or toothpaste to sink.			
12. Lined sink with towel and filled with water.			
13. Rinsed each denture under warm running water. a. Returned to denture cup.			
14. Applied denture cleaner or toothpaste to brush.			
15. Brushed dentures as in Fig. 9.			
16. Rinsed dentures under warm running water. a. Handled carefully, not dropped.			
17. Placed in denture cup. a. Filled with cool water until dentures were covered.			
18. Cleaned kidney basin.			
19. Brought denture cup and kidney basin to bedside.			
20. Raised or lowered bed rails as needed.			
21. Positioned resident for oral hygiene.			
22. Asked resident to rinse mouth with mouthwash. a. Held kidney (emesis) basin under chin.			
23. Asked resident to insert dentures.			

STEPS	S	U	COMMENTS
24. If resident unable, inserted dentures. Upper dentures: a. Grasped firmly with thumb and index finger. b. Raised upper lip with other hand and inserted denture. c. Used index fingers to press gently to make sure securely in place. Lower dentures: a. Grasped with thumb and index finger. b. Pulled down slightly on lower lip and inserted denture. c. Gently pressed to make sure in place.			
25. Put denture cup away.			
26. Removed and discarded gloves.			
27. Made resident comfortable.			
28. Placed signal light within reach.			
29. Raised or lowered side rails as necessary.			
30. Unscreened resident.			
31. Cleaned and returned equipment.			
32. Washed hands.			
33. Reported observations to nurse.			

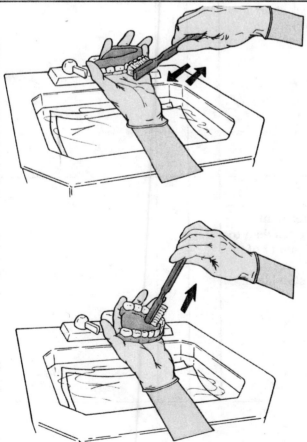

Fig. 9 Brushing dentures. (From Sorrentino SA: *Mosby's textbook for nursing assistants,* ed 4, St Louis, 1996, Mosby–Year Book.)

SKILL 26
Dressing the Resident (TNA 338–339; LTCA 272–273)

STEPS	S	U	COMMENTS
1. Identified resident. 　a. Checked ID bracelet. 　b. Called person by name.			
2. Explained procedure.			
3. Washed hands.			
4. Got a bath blanket and necessary clothing.			
5. Provided privacy.			
6. Raised the bed to the best level for good body mechanics.			
7. Undressed the resident.			
8. Covered resident with bath blanket. 　a. Fan-folded linens to foot of bed. 　b. Did not expose the resident.			
9. Lowered the side rail on the resident's strong side.			
10. Placed resident in supine position.			
Steps 11–14 are optional			
11. Put on garments that open in the back. 　a. Slid garment onto the arm and shoulder of the weak side. 　b. Slid garment onto the arm and shoulder of the strong side. 　c. Raised resident's head and shoulders. 　d. Brought sides of garment to the back. 　e. If resident in side-lying position: 　　1) Turned resident towards you. 　　2) Brought sides of garment to resident's back. 　　3) Turned resident away. 　　4) Brought other side of garment to resident's back. 　f. Fastened buttons, snaps, ties or zippers. 　g. Positioned resident in supine position.			
12. Put on garments that opened in front. 　a. Slid garment onto arm and shoulder on the weak side. 　b. Raised head and shoulders by locking arms with resident. Brought side of garment around the back. Lowered resident to supine position. Slid garment onto the arm and shoulder of the strong arm. 　c. Did following if resident unable to raise head and shoulders: 　　1) Turned resident toward you. 　　2) Tucked garment under resident. 　　3) Turned resident away. 　　4) Pulled garment out from under the resident. 　　5) Turned resident back to supine position. 　　6) Slid garment over arm and shoulder of strong arm. 　d. Fastened buttons, snaps, ties, or zippers.			

STEPS	S	U	COMMENTS

13. Put on pullover garments.
   a. Positioned resident supine.
   b. Brought neck of garment over head.
   c. Slid the arm and shoulder of garment onto the weak side.
   d. Raised resident's head and shoulders.
   e. Brought garment down.
   f. Slid arm and shoulder of garment onto strong side.
   g. Did following if resident unable to assume semi-sitting position:
     1) Turned resident towards you.
     2) Tucked garment under resident.
     3) Turned resident away.
     4) Pulled garment out from under resident.
     5) Returned resident to supine position.
     6) Slid arm and shoulder of garment onto strong side.
   h. Fastened buttons, snaps, ties, or zippers.			

14. Put on pants or slacks.
   a. Slid pants over feet and up legs.
   b. Asked resident to raise hips and buttocks off bed.
   c. Brought pants up over buttocks and hips.
   d. Asked resident to lower hips and buttocks.
   e. Did following if resident unable to raise hips and buttocks.
     1) Turned resident onto strong side.
     2) Pulled pants over buttock and hip on weak side.
     3) Turned resident on weak side.
     4) Pulled pants over buttock and hip on strong side.
     5) Positioned resident supine.
   f. Fastened buttons, ties, snaps, zipper, and belt buckle.			

15. Put socks and shoes or slippers on resident.			
16. Helped resident get out of bed if he or she wants to be up.			

17. Did following for resident who will stay in bed.
   a. Covered resident and removed bath blanket.
   b. Made sure resident was comfortable.
   c. Lowered the bed to its lowest position.
   d. Raised or lowered side rails as appropriate.
   e. Placed call light within reach.			

18. Unscreened resident.			
19. Placed soiled clothing in appropriate place.			
20. Washed hands.			
21. Reported observations to nurse.			

SKILL 27
Brushing and Combing the Resident's Hair (TNA 322; LTCA 260)

STEPS	S	U	COMMENTS

1. Identified resident.
   a. Checked ID bracelet.
   b. Called person by name.			

2. Explained procedure.			

3. Collected the following:
   a. Comb and brush
   b. Bath towel
   c. Other toilet items as requested			

4. Arranged items on the bedside stand.			
5. Washed your hands.			
6. Provided privacy.			
7. Lowered side rail if up.			
8. Helped resident to chair or semi-Fowler's position if allowed. a. Resident is dressed or has on robe and slippers.			
9. Placed towel across resident's shoulders. a. Placed towel across pillow if resident is in bed.			

10. Asked resident to remove eyeglasses.
   a. Put in glass case.
   b. Put glass case in bedside stand.			

11. Part hair into 2 main sections. a. Then divide one side into 2 sections.			
12. Brushed hair. a. Started at scalp and brushed toward the hair ends.			
13. Styled hair as the resident prefers.			
14. Removed the towel.			
15. Let resident put eyeglasses on.			
16. Assisted resident to a comfortable position.			
17. Raised or lowered bed rails as needed.			
18. Placed signal light within reach.			
19. Unscreened resident.			
20. Cleaned and returned equipment to its proper place. a. Placed soiled linen in linen hamper.			
21. Washed hands.			

SKILL 28
Giving Nail and Foot Care (TNA 329; LTCA 266)

STEPS	S	U	COMMENTS
1. Explained procedure.			
2. Washed hands.			

3. Collected necessary equipment:
  a. Wash basin
  b. Bath thermometer
  c. Bath towel
  d. Face towel
  e. Wash cloth
  f. Kidney basin
  g. Nail clippers
  h. Orange stick
  i. Emery board or nail file
  j. Lotion or petrolatum
  k. Paper towels
  l. Disposable bath mat			

4. Arranged the equipment on the overbed table.			

5. Identified resident.
  a. Checked ID bracelet.
  b. Called person by name.			

6. Provided privacy.			
7. Assisted resident to bedside chair. a. Placed signal light within reach.			
8. Placed the bath mat under resident's feet.			
9. Filled basin. a. Water temperature should be 109° F (42° C).			
10. Placed wash basin on floor on towel. a. Helped resident put feet into basin.			
11. Positioned overbed table in front of resident. a. Was low and close to resident.			
12. Filled kidney basin. a. Water temperature 109° F (42° C).			
13. Placed kidney basin on overbed table on top of paper towels.			
14. Placed resident's fingers in basin. a. Positioned arms so resident is comfortable.			
15. Soaked fingernails 15 to 20 minutes. a. Rewarmed water in 10 to 15 minutes.			
16. Cleaned under fingernails with orange stick.			
17. Removed kidney basin. a. Dried fingers thoroughly.			
18. Clipped fingernails straight across with nail clippers.			
19. Shaped nails with emery board or nail file.			
20. Pushed cuticles back with wash cloth or orange stick.			

STEPS	S	U	COMMENTS
21. Moved overbed table from in front of resident.			
22. Scrubbed callused areas of feet with wash cloth.			
23. Removed feet from basin. a. Dried thoroughly, especially between toes.			
NOTE: Nursing assistants do not cut or trim toenails.			
24. Applied lotion or petrolatum to tops and soles of feet. a. Did not apply between toes.			
25. Helped resident back to bed (if indicated) and to a comfortable position. a. Placed call light within reach.			
26. Raised or lowered side rails as instructed by nurse.			
27. Put socks and shoes or slippers on resident who will stay up.			
28. Cleaned and returned equipment and supplies to proper places. a. Discarded disposable supplies.			
29. Unscreened resident.			
30. Took soiled linen to linen hamper.			
31. Washed hands.			

32. Reported observations to nurse:
    a. Reddened, irritated, or callused areas.
    b. Breaks in skin.			

SKILL 29 Serving Meal Trays (TNA 417; LTCA 347)			
STEPS	**S**	**U**	**COMMENTS**
1. Washed hands.			
2. Checked items on tray with dietary card and made sure tray was complete.			

3. Identified resident.
  a. Checked ID bracelet with dietary card.
  b. Called person by name.			

4. Placed resident in sitting position if possible.			
5. Placed tray on overbed table or dining room table within easy reach of resident. a. Adjusted table height as necessary.			

6. Removed food covers.
  a. Opened milk cartons and cereal boxes.
  b. Cut meat, if indicated.
  c. Buttered bread, if indicated.			

7. Placed napkin and silverware within resident's reach.			
8. Measured and recorded intake, if ordered. a. Noted amount and type of foods eaten.			
9. Removed tray.			
10. Assisted resident with oral hygiene.			
11. Cleaned any spills. a. Changed soiled linen.			
12. Helped resident back to bed (if indicated) and to a comfortable position. a. Placed call light within reach.			
13. Raised or lowered side rails as instructed by nurse.			
14. Washed hands.			
15. Reported observations to nurse.			

SKILL 30 **Providing Drinking Water** (TNA 419; LTCA 350)			
STEPS	S	U	COMMENTS
1. Asked nurse for list of residents with special fluid orders (e.g. NPO, fluid restriction, no ice).			
2. Asked co-worker to assist.			
3. Washed hands.			

4. Collected the following:
  a. Cart for dirty pitchers, glasses, and trays.
  b. Cart containing clean water, pitchers, glasses and trays.
  c. Scoop for ice machine.
  d. Straws.			

5. Took cart with clean equipment to ice machine.
  a. Used scoop to put ice into water pitchers.
  b. Had helper fill pitchers with water.			

6. Rolled both carts to area just outside resident's room. a. Checked list to see if resident had special orders.			
7. Had helper take dirty pitcher, glass, and tray from resident's room. a. Placed on empty cart.			

8. Identified resident.
  a. Checked ID bracelet.
  b. Called person by name.			

9. Placed tray with pitcher, glass, and straw on overbed table. a. Made sure resident could easily reach items.			
10. Filled glass with fresh water.			
11. Repeated steps 5 through 10 for each resident.			
12. Returned cart with dirty equipment to kitchen to be washed.			
13. Washed hands.			

SKILL 31			
Giving the Bedpan (TNA 347–348; LTCA 288)			
STEPS	**S**	**U**	**COMMENTS**
1. Identified resident. a. Checked ID bracelet. b. Called person by name.			
2. Provided privacy.			
3. Collected the following: a. Bedpan b. Bedpan cover c. Toilet tissue d. Disposable gloves			
4. Arranged equipment on the chair or bed.			
5. Explained procedure to resident.			
6. Raised bed to best level for body mechanics. a. Made sure side rails are up.			
7. Put on gloves.			
8. Warmed and dried bedpan.			
9. Lowered side rail near you.			
10. Positioned resident supine. a. Elevated head of bed slightly.			
11. Folded top linens out of way. a. Kept lower portion of body covered.			
12. Asked resident to flex knees and raise buttocks by pushing against mattress with feet.			
13. Slid hand under lower back. a. Helped resident raise buttocks.			
14. Slid bedpan under resident.			
15. Did following if resident unable to assist: a. Turned resident onto side away from you. b. Placed bedpan firmly against buttocks. c. Pushed bedpan down and toward resident. d. Held bedpan securely. e. Turned resident onto back. f. Centered bedpan under resident.			
16. Returned top linens to proper position.			
17. Raised head of bed so resident in sitting position.			
18. Made sure resident correctly positioned on bedpan.			
19. Raised side rail.			
20. Placed toilet tissue and signal light within reach.			
21. Asked resident to signal when through or assistance needed.			
22. Left room and closed door. a. Washed hands.			
23. Returned when resident signaled.			

STEPS	S	U	COMMENTS
24. Lowered side rail and head of bed.			
25. Put on gloves.			

26. Asked resident to raise buttocks.
   a. Removed bedpan.
   b. Held bedpan securely and turned resident away from you (if indicated).			

27. Cleaned genital area if resident unable.
   a. Cleaned from front to back with toilet tissue.
   b. Provided perineal care if necessary.			

28. Covered bedpan.
   a. Raised side rail.
   b. Took to bathroom or "dirty" utility room.			

29. Measured urine if resident on intake and output.
   a. Collected urine specimen if needed.
   b. Noted color, amount, and character of urine or feces.			

30. Emptied and rinsed bedpan. a. Cleaned with disinfectant if indicated.			
31. Returned bedpan and clean cover to bedside stand.			
32. Removed gloves.			
33. Helped resident wash hands.			
34. Made sure resident was comfortable.			
35. Lowered bed to lowest position.			
36. Placed signal light within reach.			
37. Lowered side rails as instructed by nurse.			
38. Unscreened resident.			
39. Placed soiled linen in linen hamper.			
40. Washed hands.			
41. Reported observations to nurse.			

Index